PERSONAL INF

Name: _____

Address: _____

_____

Phone Number: _____

Date of Birth: _____

Allergies: _____

_____

Emergency Contact

Name: _____

Phone Number:_____

We are delighted you chose us to help monitor and improve your health! If you enjoy the content of this book please consider leaving a review for us on Amazon!

Your feedback helps others make the best decision for their health, too!

CONTENTS

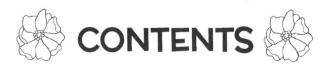

How To Use The Daily Logs

Fill in this chart for each meal and snack you enjoy throughout the day. Don't forget to total the nutritional content for each meal!

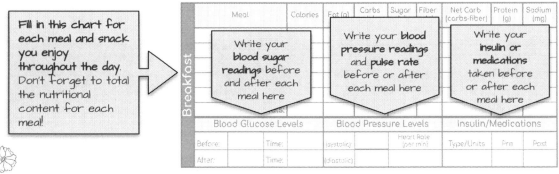

	Meal	Calories	Fat (g)	Carbs	Sugar	Fiber	Net Carb (carbs-fiber)	Protein (g)	Sodium (mg)
Breakfast									

Write your **blood sugar readings** before and after each meal here

Write your **blood pressure readings** and pulse rate before or after each meal here

Write your **insulin or medications** taken before or after each meal here

Blood Glucose Levels		Blood Pressure Levels		Insulin/Medications		
			Heart Rate (per min)	Type/Units	Pre	Post
Before:	Time:	(systolic)				
After:	Time:	(diastolic)				

Water Intake:

_____ total ounces

Record your **daily water intake.** As you drink **8oz** of water, mark off a bottle from the page!

Fitness Log:

Activity	Min

Document your **daily activities.** List the activity and duration, in minutes, the activity lasted. Fitness plays a huge part in your health!

Sleep Log:

_____ hours

Keep track of your **sleep.** Do you notice a pattern of higher fasting blood sugar levels when you get less sleep? Higher blood pressures?

REFERENCE VALUES

Blood Glucose Tests/Values

- **A1C Test**

  The A1C test measures your average blood sugar level over the past 2 or 3 months. **An A1C below 5.7% is normal**, between 5.7 and 6.4% indicates you have prediabetes, and 6.5% or higher indicates you have diabetes.

- **Fasting Blood Sugar Test**

  This measures your blood sugar after an overnight fast (not eating). **A fasting blood sugar level of 99 mg/dL or lower is normal**, 100 to 125 mg/dL indicates you have prediabetes, and 126 mg/dL or higher indicates you have diabetes.

- **Random Blood Sugar Test**

  This measures your blood sugar at the time you're tested. You can take this test at any time and don't need to fast (not eat) first. **A blood sugar level of 200 mg/dL or higher indicates you have diabetes.**

Blood Pressure Values

- **Normal**
  systolic: less than 120 mm Hg
  diastolic: less than 80 mm Hg

- **Elevated**
  systolic: 120-129 mm Hg
  diastolic: less than 80 mm Hg

- **High Blood Pressure (hypertension)**
  systolic: 130 mm Hg or higher
  diastolic: 80 mm Hg or higher

> ## The values provided are for reference only.
>
> If you have values outside of the normal range please contact your physician and/or 911 in the case of an emergency.

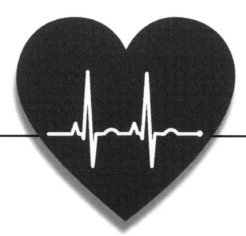

Reference testing and lab values obtained from the Center for Disease Control
https://www.cdc.gov/diabetes/basics/getting-tested.html
https://www.cdc.gov/bloodpressure/about.htm

DOCTOR APPOINTMENTS

Date:_____
Time:_____
Place:_____
Doctor:_____
Reason: _____
_____
Notes:_____
_____
_____
_____
_____
_____
_____
Next Visit:_____

Date:_____
Time:_____
Place:_____
Doctor:_____
Reason: _____
_____
Notes:_____
_____
_____
_____
_____
_____
_____
Next Visit:_____

Date:_____
Time:_____
Place:_____
Doctor:_____
Reason: _____
_____
Notes:_____
_____
_____
_____
_____
_____
_____
Next Visit:_____

Date:_____
Time:_____
Place:_____
Doctor:_____
Reason: _____
_____
Notes:_____
_____
_____
_____
_____
_____
_____
Next Visit:_____

DOCTOR APPOINTMENTS

Date:_____
Time:_____
Place:_____
Doctor:_____
Reason: _____
_____
Notes:_____
_____
_____
_____
_____
_____
_____
Next Visit:_____

Date:_____
Time:_____
Place:_____
Doctor:_____
Reason: _____
_____
Notes:_____
_____
_____
_____
_____
_____
_____
Next Visit:_____

Date:_____
Time:_____
Place:_____
Doctor:_____
Reason: _____
_____
Notes:_____
_____
_____
_____
_____
_____
_____
Next Visit:_____

Date:_____
Time:_____
Place:_____
Doctor:_____
Reason: _____
_____
Notes:_____
_____
_____
_____
_____
_____
_____
Next Visit:_____

MEDICATION LIST

Date	Name	Dosage/Directions

MEDICATION LIST

Date	Name	Dosage/Directions

WEEKLY HEALTH ANALYSIS

Weight Tracker

Date	Weight

Goal:

BMI Tracker

Date	BMI

Goal:

Hgb A1C Tracker

Date	Value

Goal:

Mood Tracker

Date	Mood (circle one)
	👍 OK 👎
	👍 OK 👎
	👍 OK 👎
	👍 OK 👎
	👍 OK 👎
	👍 OK 👎
	👍 OK 👎
	👍 OK 👎
	👍 OK 👎
	👍 OK 👎
	👍 OK 👎
	👍 OK 👎
	👍 OK 👎

Other Tests

Date	Test	Result	Notes

WEEKLY HEALTH ANALYSIS

Weight Tracker

Date	Weight

Goal:

BMI Tracker

Date	BMI

Goal:

Hgb A1C Tracker

Date	Value

Goal:

Mood Tracker

Date	Mood (circle one)
	👍 OK 👎
	👍 OK 👎
	👍 OK 👎
	👍 OK 👎
	👍 OK 👎
	👍 OK 👎
	👍 OK 👎
	👍 OK 👎
	👍 OK 👎
	👍 OK 👎
	👍 OK 👎
	👍 OK 👎
	👍 OK 👎

Other Tests

Date	Test	Result	Notes

SYMPTOMS TRACKER Month: _____

Symptom	1	2	3	4	5	6	7	8	9	10	11	12	13	14	15	16	17	18	19	20	21	22	23	24	25	26	27	28	29	30	31

Month: _____

Symptom	1	2	3	4	5	6	7	8	9	10	11	12	13	14	15	16	17	18	19	20	21	22	23	24	25	26	27	28	29	30	31

SYMPTOMS TRACKER

Month: _____

Symptom	1	2	3	4	5	6	7	8	9	10	11	12	13	14	15	16	17	18	19	20	21	22	23	24	25	26	27	28	29	30	31

Month: _____

Symptom	1	2	3	4	5	6	7	8	9	10	11	12	13	14	15	16	17	18	19	20	21	22	23	24	25	26	27	28	29	30	31

SYMPTOMS TRACKER Month: _____

Symptom	1	2	3	4	5	6	7	8	9	10	11	12	13	14	15	16	17	18	19	20	21	22	23	24	25	26	27	28	29	30	31

Month: _____

Symptom	1	2	3	4	5	6	7	8	9	10	11	12	13	14	15	16	17	18	19	20	21	22	23	24	25	26	27	28	29	30	31

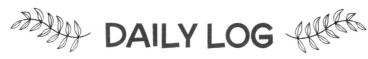

DAILY LOG

Date: ___/___/_____   **M T W Th F Sa Su**

Breakfast

Meal	Calories	Fat (g)	Carbs (g)	Sugar (g)	Fiber (g)	Net Carb (carbs-fiber)	Protein (g)	Sodium (mg)
Totals:								

Blood Glucose Levels			Blood Pressure Levels			Insulin/Medications		
Before:		Time:	(systolic):		Heart Rate (per min)	Type/Units	Pre	Post
After:		Time:	(diastolic):					

Fasting Blood Sugar:

_____

Snack #1

Meal	Calories	Fat (g)	Carbs (g)	Sugar (g)	Fiber (g)	Net Carb (carbs-fiber)	Protein (g)	Sodium (mg)
Totals:								

Blood Glucose Levels			Blood Pressure Levels			Insulin/Medications		
Before:		Time:	(systolic):		Heart Rate (per min)	Type/Units	Pre	Post
After:		Time:	(diastolic):					

Water Intake:

🍼 🍼 🍼 🍼 🍼 🍼 🍼 🍼

total ounces _____

Fitness Log:

Activity	Min

Lunch

Meal	Calories	Fat (g)	Carbs (g)	Sugar (g)	Fiber (g)	Net Carb (carbs-fiber)	Protein (g)	Sodium (mg)
Totals:								

Blood Glucose Levels			Blood Pressure Levels			Insulin/Medications		
Before:		Time:	(systolic):		Heart Rate (per min)	Type/Units	Pre	Post
After:		Time:	(diastolic):					

Sleep Log:

Total Hours _____

Snack #2

Meal	Calories	Fat (g)	Carbs (g)	Sugar (g)	Fiber (g)	Net Carb (carbs-fiber)	Protein (g)	Sodium (mg)
Totals:								

Blood Glucose Levels			Blood Pressure Levels			Insulin/Medications		
Before:		Time:	(systolic):		Heart Rate (per min)	Type/Units	Pre	Post
After:		Time:	(diastolic):					

Notes:

_____
_____
_____
_____
_____
_____

Dinner

Meal	Calories	Fat (g)	Carbs (g)	Sugar (g)	Fiber (g)	Net Carb (carbs-fiber)	Protein (g)	Sodium (mg)
Totals:								

Blood Glucose Levels			Blood Pressure Levels			Insulin/Medications		
Before:		Time:	(systolic):		Heart Rate (per min)	Type/Units	Pre	Post
After:		Time:	(diastolic):					

DAILY LOG

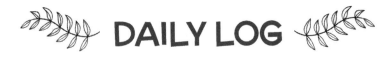

Date: ___/___/_____   **M T W Th F Sa Su**

Breakfast

Meal	Calories	Fat (g)	Carbs (g)	Sugar (g)	Fiber (g)	Net Carb (carbs-fiber)	Protein (g)	Sodium (mg)
Totals:								

Blood Glucose Levels				Blood Pressure Levels			Insulin/Medications		
Before:		Time:		(systolic):		Heart Rate (per min)	Type/Units	Pre	Post
After:		Time:		(diastolic):					

Snack #1

Meal	Calories	Fat (g)	Carbs (g)	Sugar (g)	Fiber (g)	Net Carb (carbs-fiber)	Protein (g)	Sodium (mg)
Totals:								

Blood Glucose Levels				Blood Pressure Levels			Insulin/Medications		
Before:		Time:		(systolic):		Heart Rate (per min)	Type/Units	Pre	Post
After:		Time:		(diastolic):					

Lunch

Meal	Calories	Fat (g)	Carbs (g)	Sugar (g)	Fiber (g)	Net Carb (carbs-fiber)	Protein (g)	Sodium (mg)
Totals:								

Blood Glucose Levels				Blood Pressure Levels			Insulin/Medications		
Before:		Time:		(systolic):		Heart Rate (per min)	Type/Units	Pre	Post
After:		Time:		(diastolic):					

Snack #2

Meal	Calories	Fat (g)	Carbs (g)	Sugar (g)	Fiber (g)	Net Carb (carbs-fiber)	Protein (g)	Sodium (mg)
Totals:								

Blood Glucose Levels				Blood Pressure Levels			Insulin/Medications		
Before:		Time:		(systolic):		Heart Rate (per min)	Type/Units	Pre	Post
After:		Time:		(diastolic):					

Dinner

Meal	Calories	Fat (g)	Carbs (g)	Sugar (g)	Fiber (g)	Net Carb (carbs-fiber)	Protein (g)	Sodium (mg)
Totals:								

Blood Glucose Levels				Blood Pressure Levels			Insulin/Medications		
Before:		Time:		(systolic):		Heart Rate (per min)	Type/Units	Pre	Post
After:		Time:		(diastolic):					

Fasting Blood Sugar:

_____

Water Intake:

total ounces _____

Fitness Log:

Activity	Min

Sleep Log:

Total Hours _____

Notes:

_____
_____
_____
_____
_____
_____
_____
_____

DAILY LOG

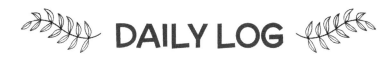

Date: ___/___/_____

M T W Th F Sa Su

Breakfast

Meal	Calories	Fat (g)	Carbs (g)	Sugar (g)	Fiber (g)	Net Carb (carbs-fiber)	Protein (g)	Sodium (mg)
Totals:								

Blood Glucose Levels			Blood Pressure Levels		Insulin/Medications		
Before:		Time:	(systolic):	Heart Rate (per min)	Type/Units	Pre	Post
After:		Time:	(diastolic):				

Snack #1

Totals:								

Blood Glucose Levels			Blood Pressure Levels		Insulin/Medications		
Before:		Time:	(systolic):	Heart Rate (per min)	Type/Units	Pre	Post
After:		Time:	(diastolic):				

Lunch

Totals:								

Blood Glucose Levels			Blood Pressure Levels		Insulin/Medications		
Before:		Time:	(systolic):	Heart Rate (per min)	Type/Units	Pre	Post
After:		Time:	(diastolic):				

Snack #2

Totals:								

Blood Glucose Levels			Blood Pressure Levels		Insulin/Medications		
Before:		Time:	(systolic):	Heart Rate (per min)	Type/Units	Pre	Post
After:		Time:	(diastolic):				

Dinner

Totals:								

Blood Glucose Levels			Blood Pressure Levels		Insulin/Medications		
Before:		Time:	(systolic):	Heart Rate (per min)	Type/Units	Pre	Post
After:		Time:	(diastolic):				

Fasting Blood Sugar:

_____

Water Intake:

total ounces _____

Fitness Log:

Activity	Min

Sleep Log:

Total Hours _____

Notes:

_____
_____
_____
_____
_____
_____
_____
_____
_____
_____

DAILY LOG

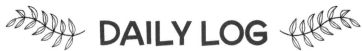

Date: _____/_____/_____   **M T W Th F Sa Su**

Breakfast

	Meal	Calories	Fat (g)	Carbs (g)	Sugar (g)	Fiber (g)	Net Carb (carbs-fiber)	Protein (g)	Sodium (mg)
	Totals:								

Blood Glucose Levels				Blood Pressure Levels			Insulin/Medications		
Before:		Time:		(systolic):		Heart Rate (per min)	Type/Units	Pre	Post
After:		Time:		(diastolic):					

Snack #1

	Totals:								

Blood Glucose Levels				Blood Pressure Levels			Insulin/Medications		
Before:		Time:		(systolic):		Heart Rate (per min)	Type/Units	Pre	Post
After:		Time:		(diastolic):					

Lunch

	Totals:								

Blood Glucose Levels				Blood Pressure Levels			Insulin/Medications		
Before:		Time:		(systolic):		Heart Rate (per min)	Type/Units	Pre	Post
After:		Time:		(diastolic):					

Snack #2

	Totals:								

Blood Glucose Levels				Blood Pressure Levels			Insulin/Medications		
Before:		Time:		(systolic):		Heart Rate (per min)	Type/Units	Pre	Post
After:		Time:		(diastolic):					

Dinner

	Totals:								

Blood Glucose Levels				Blood Pressure Levels			Insulin/Medications		
Before:		Time:		(systolic):		Heart Rate (per min)	Type/Units	Pre	Post
After:		Time:		(diastolic):					

Fasting Blood Sugar:

_____

Water Intake:

total ounces _____

Fitness Log:

Activity	Min

Sleep Log:

Total Hours _____

Notes:

DAILY LOG

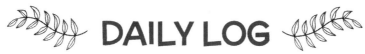

Date: ____/____/_____   **M   T   W   Th   F   Sa   Su**

Breakfast

Meal	Calories	Fat (g)	Carbs (g)	Sugar (g)	Fiber (g)	Net Carb (carbs-fiber)	Protein (g)	Sodium (mg)
Totals:								

Blood Glucose Levels		Blood Pressure Levels		Insulin/Medications		
Before:	Time:	(systolic):	Heart Rate (per min)	Type/Units	Pre	Post
After:	Time:	(diastolic):				

Snack #1

Meal	Calories	Fat (g)	Carbs (g)	Sugar (g)	Fiber (g)	Net Carb (carbs-fiber)	Protein (g)	Sodium (mg)
Totals:								

Blood Glucose Levels		Blood Pressure Levels		Insulin/Medications		
Before:	Time:	(systolic):	Heart Rate (per min)	Type/Units	Pre	Post
After:	Time:	(diastolic):				

Lunch

Meal	Calories	Fat (g)	Carbs (g)	Sugar (g)	Fiber (g)	Net Carb (carbs-fiber)	Protein (g)	Sodium (mg)
Totals:								

Blood Glucose Levels		Blood Pressure Levels		Insulin/Medications		
Before:	Time:	(systolic):	Heart Rate (per min)	Type/Units	Pre	Post
After:	Time:	(diastolic):				

Snack #2

Meal	Calories	Fat (g)	Carbs (g)	Sugar (g)	Fiber (g)	Net Carb (carbs-fiber)	Protein (g)	Sodium (mg)
Totals:								

Blood Glucose Levels		Blood Pressure Levels		Insulin/Medications		
Before:	Time:	(systolic):	Heart Rate (per min)	Type/Units	Pre	Post
After:	Time:	(diastolic):				

Dinner

Meal	Calories	Fat (g)	Carbs (g)	Sugar (g)	Fiber (g)	Net Carb (carbs-fiber)	Protein (g)	Sodium (mg)
Totals:								

Blood Glucose Levels		Blood Pressure Levels		Insulin/Medications		
Before:	Time:	(systolic):	Heart Rate (per min)	Type/Units	Pre	Post
After:	Time:	(diastolic):				

Fasting Blood Sugar:

_____

Water Intake:

total ounces _____

Fitness Log:

Activity	Min

Sleep Log:

Total Hours _____

Notes:

DAILY LOG

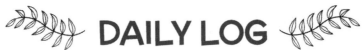

Date: ___/___/_____

M T W Th F Sa Su

Breakfast

Meal	Calories	Fat (g)	Carbs (g)	Sugar (g)	Fiber (g)	Net Carb (carbs-fiber)	Protein (g)	Sodium (mg)
Totals:								

Blood Glucose Levels			Blood Pressure Levels		Insulin/Medications		
Before:		Time:	(systolic):	Heart Rate (per min)	Type/Units	Pre	Post
After:		Time:	(diastolic):				

Snack #1

	Calories	Fat (g)	Carbs (g)	Sugar (g)	Fiber (g)	Net Carb (carbs-fiber)	Protein (g)	Sodium (mg)
Totals:								

Blood Glucose Levels			Blood Pressure Levels		Insulin/Medications		
Before:		Time:	(systolic):	Heart Rate (per min)	Type/Units	Pre	Post
After:		Time:	(diastolic):				

Lunch

	Calories	Fat (g)	Carbs (g)	Sugar (g)	Fiber (g)	Net Carb (carbs-fiber)	Protein (g)	Sodium (mg)
Totals:								

Blood Glucose Levels			Blood Pressure Levels		Insulin/Medications		
Before:		Time:	(systolic):	Heart Rate (per min)	Type/Units	Pre	Post
After:		Time:	(diastolic):				

Snack #2

	Calories	Fat (g)	Carbs (g)	Sugar (g)	Fiber (g)	Net Carb (carbs-fiber)	Protein (g)	Sodium (mg)
Totals:								

Blood Glucose Levels			Blood Pressure Levels		Insulin/Medications		
Before:		Time:	(systolic):	Heart Rate (per min)	Type/Units	Pre	Post
After:		Time:	(diastolic):				

Dinner

	Calories	Fat (g)	Carbs (g)	Sugar (g)	Fiber (g)	Net Carb (carbs-fiber)	Protein (g)	Sodium (mg)
Totals:								

Blood Glucose Levels			Blood Pressure Levels		Insulin/Medications		
Before:		Time:	(systolic):	Heart Rate (per min)	Type/Units	Pre	Post
After:		Time:	(diastolic):				

Fasting Blood Sugar:

_____

Water Intake:

🍶 🍶 🍶 🍶 🍶 🍶 🍶 🍶

total ounces _____

Fitness Log:

Activity   Min

Sleep Log:

Total Hours _____

Notes:

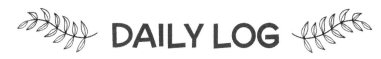

DAILY LOG

Date: ___/___/_____   M T W Th F Sa Su

Breakfast

Meal	Calories	Fat (g)	Carbs (g)	Sugar (g)	Fiber (g)	Net Carb (carbs-fiber)	Protein (g)	Sodium (mg)
Totals:								

Blood Glucose Levels		Blood Pressure Levels		Insulin/Medications		
Before:	Time:	(systolic):	Heart Rate (per min)	Type/Units	Pre	Post
After:	Time:	(diastolic):				

Snack #1

Totals:								

Blood Glucose Levels		Blood Pressure Levels		Insulin/Medications		
Before:	Time:	(systolic):	Heart Rate (per min)	Type/Units	Pre	Post
After:	Time:	(diastolic):				

Lunch

Totals:								

Blood Glucose Levels		Blood Pressure Levels		Insulin/Medications		
Before:	Time:	(systolic):	Heart Rate (per min)	Type/Units	Pre	Post
After:	Time:	(diastolic):				

Snack #2

Totals:								

Blood Glucose Levels		Blood Pressure Levels		Insulin/Medications		
Before:	Time:	(systolic):	Heart Rate (per min)	Type/Units	Pre	Post
After:	Time:	(diastolic):				

Dinner

Totals:								

Blood Glucose Levels		Blood Pressure Levels		Insulin/Medications		
Before:	Time:	(systolic):	Heart Rate (per min)	Type/Units	Pre	Post
After:	Time:	(diastolic):				

Fasting Blood Sugar:

_____

Water Intake:

total ounces _____

Fitness Log:

Activity	Min

Sleep Log:

Total Hours _____

Notes:

_____
_____
_____
_____
_____
_____
_____
_____
_____
_____
_____
_____

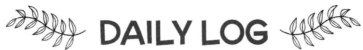

DAILY LOG

Date: ___/___/_____   M T W Th F Sa Su

Breakfast

Meal	Calories	Fat (g)	Carbs (g)	Sugar (g)	Fiber (g)	Net Carb (carbs-fiber)	Protein (g)	Sodium (mg)
Totals:								

Blood Glucose Levels				Blood Pressure Levels			Insulin/Medications		
Before:		Time:		(systolic):		Heart Rate (per min)	Type/Units	Pre	Post
After:		Time:		(diastolic):					

Snack #1

Totals:								

Blood Glucose Levels				Blood Pressure Levels			Insulin/Medications		
Before:		Time:		(systolic):		Heart Rate (per min)	Type/Units	Pre	Post
After:		Time:		(diastolic):					

Lunch

Totals:								

Blood Glucose Levels				Blood Pressure Levels			Insulin/Medications		
Before:		Time:		(systolic):		Heart Rate (per min)	Type/Units	Pre	Post
After:		Time:		(diastolic):					

Snack #2

Totals:								

Blood Glucose Levels				Blood Pressure Levels			Insulin/Medications		
Before:		Time:		(systolic):		Heart Rate (per min)	Type/Units	Pre	Post
After:		Time:		(diastolic):					

Dinner

Totals:								

Blood Glucose Levels				Blood Pressure Levels			Insulin/Medications		
Before:		Time:		(systolic):		Heart Rate (per min)	Type/Units	Pre	Post
After:		Time:		(diastolic):					

Fasting Blood Sugar:
_____

Water Intake:
total ounces _____

Fitness Log:

Activity	Min

Sleep Log:
Total Hours _____

Notes:

DAILY LOG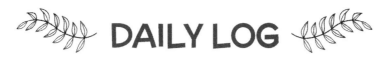

Date: ___/___/_____   **M T W Th F Sa Su**

Breakfast

	Meal	Calories	Fat (g)	Carbs (g)	Sugar (g)	Fiber (g)	Net Carb (carbs-fiber)	Protein (g)	Sodium (mg)
	Totals:								

Blood Glucose Levels			Blood Pressure Levels			Insulin/Medications		
Before:		Time:	(systolic):		Heart Rate (per min)	Type/Units	Pre	Post
After:		Time:	(diastolic):					

Snack #1

	Totals:								

Blood Glucose Levels			Blood Pressure Levels			Insulin/Medications		
Before:		Time:	(systolic):		Heart Rate (per min)	Type/Units	Pre	Post
After:		Time:	(diastolic):					

Lunch

	Totals:								

Blood Glucose Levels			Blood Pressure Levels			Insulin/Medications		
Before:		Time:	(systolic):		Heart Rate (per min)	Type/Units	Pre	Post
After:		Time:	(diastolic):					

Snack #2

	Totals:								

Blood Glucose Levels			Blood Pressure Levels			Insulin/Medications		
Before:		Time:	(systolic):		Heart Rate (per min)	Type/Units	Pre	Post
After:		Time:	(diastolic):					

Dinner

	Totals:								

Blood Glucose Levels			Blood Pressure Levels			Insulin/Medications		
Before:		Time:	(systolic):		Heart Rate (per min)	Type/Units	Pre	Post
After:		Time:	(diastolic):					

Fasting Blood Sugar:
_____

Water Intake:
🍶 🍶 🍶 🍶 🍶 🍶 🍶 🍶
total ounces _____

Fitness Log:

Activity	Min

Sleep Log:
Total Hours _____

Notes:
_____
_____
_____
_____
_____
_____
_____
_____
_____

DAILY LOG

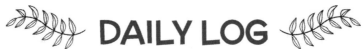

Date: ___/___/_____   **M T W Th F Sa Su**

Breakfast

Meal	Calories	Fat (g)	Carbs (g)	Sugar (g)	Fiber (g)	Net Carb (carbs-fiber)	Protein (g)	Sodium (mg)
Totals:								

Blood Glucose Levels				Blood Pressure Levels			Insulin/Medications		
Before:		Time:		(systolic):		Heart Rate (per min)	Type/Units	Pre	Post
After:		Time:		(diastolic):					

Snack #1

Totals:									

Blood Glucose Levels				Blood Pressure Levels			Insulin/Medications		
Before:		Time:		(systolic):		Heart Rate (per min)	Type/Units	Pre	Post
After:		Time:		(diastolic):					

Lunch

Totals:									

Blood Glucose Levels				Blood Pressure Levels			Insulin/Medications		
Before:		Time:		(systolic):		Heart Rate (per min)	Type/Units	Pre	Post
After:		Time:		(diastolic):					

Snack #2

Totals:									

Blood Glucose Levels				Blood Pressure Levels			Insulin/Medications		
Before:		Time:		(systolic):		Heart Rate (per min)	Type/Units	Pre	Post
After:		Time:		(diastolic):					

Dinner

Totals:									

Blood Glucose Levels				Blood Pressure Levels			Insulin/Medications		
Before:		Time:		(systolic):		Heart Rate (per min)	Type/Units	Pre	Post
After:		Time:		(diastolic):					

Fasting Blood Sugar:

_____

Water Intake:

total ounces _____

Fitness Log:

Activity   Min

Sleep Log:

Total Hours _____

Notes:

DAILY LOG

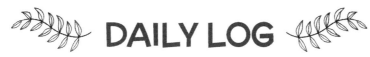

Date: ____/____/_____   **M   T   W   Th   F   Sa   Su**

Breakfast

	Meal	Calories	Fat (g)	Carbs (g)	Sugar (g)	Fiber (g)	Net Carb (carbs-fiber)	Protein (g)	Sodium (mg)
	Totals:								

Blood Glucose Levels			Blood Pressure Levels			Insulin/Medications		
Before:		Time:	(systolic):		Heart Rate (per min)	Type/Units	Pre	Post
After:		Time:	(diastolic):					

Snack #1

	Totals:								

Blood Glucose Levels			Blood Pressure Levels			Insulin/Medications		
Before:		Time:	(systolic):		Heart Rate (per min)	Type/Units	Pre	Post
After:		Time:	(diastolic):					

Lunch

	Totals:								

Blood Glucose Levels			Blood Pressure Levels			Insulin/Medications		
Before:		Time:	(systolic):		Heart Rate (per min)	Type/Units	Pre	Post
After:		Time:	(diastolic):					

Snack #2

	Totals:								

Blood Glucose Levels			Blood Pressure Levels			Insulin/Medications		
Before:		Time:	(systolic):		Heart Rate (per min)	Type/Units	Pre	Post
After:		Time:	(diastolic):					

Dinner

	Totals:								

Blood Glucose Levels			Blood Pressure Levels			Insulin/Medications		
Before:		Time:	(systolic):		Heart Rate (per min)	Type/Units	Pre	Post
After:		Time:	(diastolic):					

Fasting Blood Sugar:
_____

Water Intake:
🍼 🍼 🍼 🍼 🍼 🍼 🍼 🍼

total ounces _____

Fitness Log:

Activity	Min

Sleep Log:

Total Hours _____

Notes:
_____
_____
_____
_____
_____
_____
_____
_____
_____
_____
_____

DAILY LOG

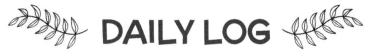

Date: ___/___/_____   **M T W Th F Sa Su**

	Meal	Calories	Fat (g)	Carbs (g)	Sugar (g)	Fiber (g)	Net Carb (carbs-fiber)	Protein (g)	Sodium (mg)
Breakfast									
	Totals:								

Breakfast

Blood Glucose Levels				Blood Pressure Levels			Insulin/Medications		
Before:		Time:		(systolic):		Heart Rate (per min)	Type/Units	Pre	Post
After:		Time:		(diastolic):					

Snack #1

	Meal	Calories	Fat (g)	Carbs (g)	Sugar (g)	Fiber (g)	Net Carb (carbs-fiber)	Protein (g)	Sodium (mg)
	Totals:								

Blood Glucose Levels				Blood Pressure Levels			Insulin/Medications		
Before:		Time:		(systolic):		Heart Rate (per min)	Type/Units	Pre	Post
After:		Time:		(diastolic):					

Lunch

	Meal	Calories	Fat (g)	Carbs (g)	Sugar (g)	Fiber (g)	Net Carb (carbs-fiber)	Protein (g)	Sodium (mg)
	Totals:								

Blood Glucose Levels				Blood Pressure Levels			Insulin/Medications		
Before:		Time:		(systolic):		Heart Rate (per min)	Type/Units	Pre	Post
After:		Time:		(diastolic):					

Snack #2

	Meal	Calories	Fat (g)	Carbs (g)	Sugar (g)	Fiber (g)	Net Carb (carbs-fiber)	Protein (g)	Sodium (mg)
	Totals:								

Blood Glucose Levels				Blood Pressure Levels			Insulin/Medications		
Before:		Time:		(systolic):		Heart Rate (per min)	Type/Units	Pre	Post
After:		Time:		(diastolic):					

Dinner

	Meal	Calories	Fat (g)	Carbs (g)	Sugar (g)	Fiber (g)	Net Carb (carbs-fiber)	Protein (g)	Sodium (mg)
	Totals:								

Blood Glucose Levels				Blood Pressure Levels			Insulin/Medications		
Before:		Time:		(systolic):		Heart Rate (per min)	Type/Units	Pre	Post
After:		Time:		(diastolic):					

Fasting Blood Sugar:

_____

Water Intake:

total ounces _____

Fitness Log:

Activity	Min

Sleep Log:

Total Hours _____

Notes:

DAILY LOG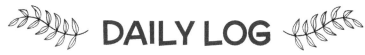

Date: ___/___/_____   M T W Th F Sa Su

Breakfast

Meal	Calories	Fat (g)	Carbs (g)	Sugar (g)	Fiber (g)	Net Carb (carbs-fiber)	Protein (g)	Sodium (mg)
Totals:								

Blood Glucose Levels		Blood Pressure Levels		Insulin/Medications		
			Heart Rate (per min)	Type/Units	Pre	Post
Before:	Time:	(systolic):				
After:	Time:	(diastolic):				

Snack #1

Totals:								

Blood Glucose Levels		Blood Pressure Levels		Insulin/Medications		
			Heart Rate (per min)	Type/Units	Pre	Post
Before:	Time:	(systolic):				
After:	Time:	(diastolic):				

Lunch

Totals:								

Blood Glucose Levels		Blood Pressure Levels		Insulin/Medications		
			Heart Rate (per min)	Type/Units	Pre	Post
Before:	Time:	(systolic):				
After:	Time:	(diastolic):				

Snack #2

Totals:								

Blood Glucose Levels		Blood Pressure Levels		Insulin/Medications		
			Heart Rate (per min)	Type/Units	Pre	Post
Before:	Time:	(systolic):				
After:	Time:	(diastolic):				

Dinner

Totals:								

Blood Glucose Levels		Blood Pressure Levels		Insulin/Medications		
			Heart Rate (per min)	Type/Units	Pre	Post
Before:	Time:	(systolic):				
After:	Time:	(diastolic):				

Fasting Blood Sugar:

_____

Water Intake:

total ounces _____

Fitness Log:

Activity	Min

Sleep Log:

Total Hours _____

Notes:

_____
_____
_____
_____
_____
_____
_____
_____

DAILY LOG
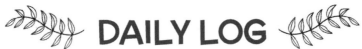

Date: ___/___/_____   **M T W Th F Sa Su**

Breakfast

Meal	Calories	Fat (g)	Carbs (g)	Sugar (g)	Fiber (g)	Net Carb (carbs-fiber)	Protein (g)	Sodium (mg)
Totals:								

Blood Glucose Levels				Blood Pressure Levels			Insulin/Medications		
Before:		Time:		(systolic):		Heart Rate (per min)	Type/Units	Pre	Post
After:		Time:		(diastolic):					

Snack #1

Totals:								

Blood Glucose Levels				Blood Pressure Levels			Insulin/Medications		
Before:		Time:		(systolic):		Heart Rate (per min)	Type/Units	Pre	Post
After:		Time:		(diastolic):					

Lunch

Totals:								

Blood Glucose Levels				Blood Pressure Levels			Insulin/Medications		
Before:		Time:		(systolic):		Heart Rate (per min)	Type/Units	Pre	Post
After:		Time:		(diastolic):					

Snack #2

Totals:								

Blood Glucose Levels				Blood Pressure Levels			Insulin/Medications		
Before:		Time:		(systolic):		Heart Rate (per min)	Type/Units	Pre	Post
After:		Time:		(diastolic):					

Dinner

Totals:								

Blood Glucose Levels				Blood Pressure Levels			Insulin/Medications		
Before:		Time:		(systolic):		Heart Rate (per min)	Type/Units	Pre	Post
After:		Time:		(diastolic):					

Fasting Blood Sugar:

_____

Water Intake:

🍼 🍼 🍼 🍼 🍼 🍼 🍼 🍼

total ounces _____

Fitness Log:

Activity	Min

Sleep Log:

Total Hours _____

Notes:

_____
_____
_____
_____
_____
_____
_____
_____
_____
_____

DAILY LOG

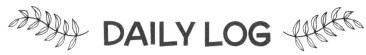

Date: ___/___/_____   **M T W Th F Sa Su**

	Meal	Calories	Fat (g)	Carbs (g)	Sugar (g)	Fiber (g)	Net Carb (carbs-fiber)	Protein (g)	Sodium (mg)
Breakfast									
	Totals:								

Blood Glucose Levels			Blood Pressure Levels		Insulin/Medications		
Before:		Time:	(systolic):	Heart Rate (per min)	Type/Units	Pre	Post
After:		Time:	(diastolic):				

		Calories	Fat (g)	Carbs (g)	Sugar (g)	Fiber (g)	Net Carb (carbs-fiber)	Protein (g)	Sodium (mg)
Snack #1									
	Totals:								

Blood Glucose Levels			Blood Pressure Levels		Insulin/Medications		
Before:		Time:	(systolic):	Heart Rate (per min)	Type/Units	Pre	Post
After:		Time:	(diastolic):				

		Calories	Fat (g)	Carbs (g)	Sugar (g)	Fiber (g)	Net Carb (carbs-fiber)	Protein (g)	Sodium (mg)
Lunch									
	Totals:								

Blood Glucose Levels			Blood Pressure Levels		Insulin/Medications		
Before:		Time:	(systolic):	Heart Rate (per min)	Type/Units	Pre	Post
After:		Time:	(diastolic):				

		Calories	Fat (g)	Carbs (g)	Sugar (g)	Fiber (g)	Net Carb (carbs-fiber)	Protein (g)	Sodium (mg)
Snack #2									
	Totals:								

Blood Glucose Levels			Blood Pressure Levels		Insulin/Medications		
Before:		Time:	(systolic):	Heart Rate (per min)	Type/Units	Pre	Post
After:		Time:	(diastolic):				

		Calories	Fat (g)	Carbs (g)	Sugar (g)	Fiber (g)	Net Carb (carbs-fiber)	Protein (g)	Sodium (mg)
Dinner									
	Totals:								

Blood Glucose Levels			Blood Pressure Levels		Insulin/Medications		
Before:		Time:	(systolic):	Heart Rate (per min)	Type/Units	Pre	Post
After:		Time:	(diastolic):				

Fasting Blood Sugar:
_____

Water Intake:
total ounces _____

Fitness Log:

Activity	Min

Sleep Log:
Total Hours _____

Notes:

DAILY LOG

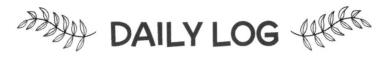

Date: ___/___/_____   **M T W Th F Sa Su**

Breakfast

Meal	Calories	Fat (g)	Carbs (g)	Sugar (g)	Fiber (g)	Net Carb (carbs-fiber)	Protein (g)	Sodium (mg)
Totals:								

Blood Glucose Levels			Blood Pressure Levels		Insulin/Medications		
Before:		Time:	(systolic):	Heart Rate (per min)	Type/Units	Pre	Post
After:		Time:	(diastolic):				

Snack #1

Meal	Calories	Fat (g)	Carbs (g)	Sugar (g)	Fiber (g)	Net Carb (carbs-fiber)	Protein (g)	Sodium (mg)
Totals:								

Blood Glucose Levels			Blood Pressure Levels		Insulin/Medications		
Before:		Time:	(systolic):	Heart Rate (per min)	Type/Units	Pre	Post
After:		Time:	(diastolic):				

Lunch

Meal	Calories	Fat (g)	Carbs (g)	Sugar (g)	Fiber (g)	Net Carb (carbs-fiber)	Protein (g)	Sodium (mg)
Totals:								

Blood Glucose Levels			Blood Pressure Levels		Insulin/Medications		
Before:		Time:	(systolic):	Heart Rate (per min)	Type/Units	Pre	Post
After:		Time:	(diastolic):				

Snack #2

Meal	Calories	Fat (g)	Carbs (g)	Sugar (g)	Fiber (g)	Net Carb (carbs-fiber)	Protein (g)	Sodium (mg)
Totals:								

Blood Glucose Levels			Blood Pressure Levels		Insulin/Medications		
Before:		Time:	(systolic):	Heart Rate (per min)	Type/Units	Pre	Post
After:		Time:	(diastolic):				

Dinner

Meal	Calories	Fat (g)	Carbs (g)	Sugar (g)	Fiber (g)	Net Carb (carbs-fiber)	Protein (g)	Sodium (mg)
Totals:								

Blood Glucose Levels			Blood Pressure Levels		Insulin/Medications		
Before:		Time:	(systolic):	Heart Rate (per min)	Type/Units	Pre	Post
After:		Time:	(diastolic):				

Fasting Blood Sugar:
_____

Water Intake:
total ounces _____

Fitness Log:

Activity	Min

Sleep Log:
Total Hours _____

Notes:
_____
_____
_____
_____
_____
_____
_____
_____
_____
_____

DAILY LOG

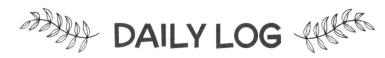

Date: ___/___/_____   **M T W Th F Sa Su**

Breakfast

Meal	Calories	Fat (g)	Carbs (g)	Sugar (g)	Fiber (g)	Net Carb (carbs-fiber)	Protein (g)	Sodium (mg)
Totals:								

Blood Glucose Levels			Blood Pressure Levels		Insulin/Medications		
Before:		Time:	(systolic):	Heart Rate (per min)	Type/Units	Pre	Post
After:		Time:	(diastolic):				

Snack #1

Totals:								

Blood Glucose Levels			Blood Pressure Levels		Insulin/Medications		
Before:		Time:	(systolic):	Heart Rate (per min)	Type/Units	Pre	Post
After:		Time:	(diastolic):				

Lunch

Totals:								

Blood Glucose Levels			Blood Pressure Levels		Insulin/Medications		
Before:		Time:	(systolic):	Heart Rate (per min)	Type/Units	Pre	Post
After:		Time:	(diastolic):				

Snack #2

Totals:								

Blood Glucose Levels			Blood Pressure Levels		Insulin/Medications		
Before:		Time:	(systolic):	Heart Rate (per min)	Type/Units	Pre	Post
After:		Time:	(diastolic):				

Dinner

Totals:								

Blood Glucose Levels			Blood Pressure Levels		Insulin/Medications		
Before:		Time:	(systolic):	Heart Rate (per min)	Type/Units	Pre	Post
After:		Time:	(diastolic):				

Fasting Blood Sugar:
_____

Water Intake:
total ounces _____

Fitness Log:

Activity	Min

Sleep Log:
Total Hours _____

Notes:
_____
_____
_____
_____
_____
_____
_____
_____
_____

DAILY LOG

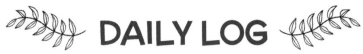

Date: ___/___/_____   M T W Th F Sa Su

Breakfast

Meal	Calories	Fat (g)	Carbs (g)	Sugar (g)	Fiber (g)	Net Carb (carbs-fiber)	Protein (g)	Sodium (mg)
Totals:								

Blood Glucose Levels				Blood Pressure Levels			Insulin/Medications		
Before:		Time:		(systolic):		Heart Rate (per min)	Type/Units	Pre	Post
After:		Time:		(diastolic):					

Snack #1

Totals:								

Blood Glucose Levels				Blood Pressure Levels			Insulin/Medications		
Before:		Time:		(systolic):		Heart Rate (per min)	Type/Units	Pre	Post
After:		Time:		(diastolic):					

Lunch

Totals:								

Blood Glucose Levels				Blood Pressure Levels			Insulin/Medications		
Before:		Time:		(systolic):		Heart Rate (per min)	Type/Units	Pre	Post
After:		Time:		(diastolic):					

Snack #2

Totals:								

Blood Glucose Levels				Blood Pressure Levels			Insulin/Medications		
Before:		Time:		(systolic):		Heart Rate (per min)	Type/Units	Pre	Post
After:		Time:		(diastolic):					

Dinner

Totals:								

Blood Glucose Levels				Blood Pressure Levels			Insulin/Medications		
Before:		Time:		(systolic):		Heart Rate (per min)	Type/Units	Pre	Post
After:		Time:		(diastolic):					

Fasting Blood Sugar:

_____

Water Intake:

total ounces _____

Fitness Log:

Activity	Min

Sleep Log:

Total Hours _____

Notes:

DAILY LOG

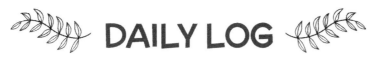

Date: ___/___/_____   **M T W Th F Sa Su**

Breakfast

	Meal	Calories	Fat (g)	Carbs (g)	Sugar (g)	Fiber (g)	Net Carb (carbs-fiber)	Protein (g)	Sodium (mg)
	Totals:								

Blood Glucose Levels			Blood Pressure Levels		Insulin/Medications		
Before:		Time:	(systolic):	Heart Rate (per min)	Type/Units	Pre	Post
After:		Time:	(diastolic):				

Snack #1

	Totals:								

Blood Glucose Levels			Blood Pressure Levels		Insulin/Medications		
Before:		Time:	(systolic):	Heart Rate (per min)	Type/Units	Pre	Post
After:		Time:	(diastolic):				

Lunch

	Totals:								

Blood Glucose Levels			Blood Pressure Levels		Insulin/Medications		
Before:		Time:	(systolic):	Heart Rate (per min)	Type/Units	Pre	Post
After:		Time:	(diastolic):				

Snack #2

	Totals:								

Blood Glucose Levels			Blood Pressure Levels		Insulin/Medications		
Before:		Time:	(systolic):	Heart Rate (per min)	Type/Units	Pre	Post
After:		Time:	(diastolic):				

Dinner

	Totals:								

Blood Glucose Levels			Blood Pressure Levels		Insulin/Medications		
Before:		Time:	(systolic):	Heart Rate (per min)	Type/Units	Pre	Post
After:		Time:	(diastolic):				

Fasting Blood Sugar:

_____

Water Intake:

total ounces _____

Fitness Log:

Activity	Min

Sleep Log:

Total Hours _____

Notes:

_____
_____
_____
_____
_____
_____
_____
_____
_____
_____

DAILY LOG

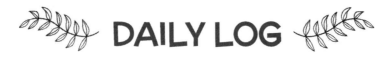

Date: ___/___/_____   **M T W Th F Sa Su**

Breakfast

	Meal	Calories	Fat (g)	Carbs (g)	Sugar (g)	Fiber (g)	Net Carb (carbs-fiber)	Protein (g)	Sodium (mg)
	Totals:								

Blood Glucose Levels				Blood Pressure Levels		Insulin/Medications		
Before:		Time:		(systolic):	Heart Rate (per min)	Type/Units	Pre	Post
After:		Time:		(diastolic):				

Snack #1

	Totals:								

Blood Glucose Levels				Blood Pressure Levels		Insulin/Medications		
Before:		Time:		(systolic):	Heart Rate (per min)	Type/Units	Pre	Post
After:		Time:		(diastolic):				

Lunch

	Totals:								

Blood Glucose Levels				Blood Pressure Levels		Insulin/Medications		
Before:		Time:		(systolic):	Heart Rate (per min)	Type/Units	Pre	Post
After:		Time:		(diastolic):				

Snack #2

	Totals:								

Blood Glucose Levels				Blood Pressure Levels		Insulin/Medications		
Before:		Time:		(systolic):	Heart Rate (per min)	Type/Units	Pre	Post
After:		Time:		(diastolic):				

Dinner

	Totals:								

Blood Glucose Levels				Blood Pressure Levels		Insulin/Medications		
Before:		Time:		(systolic):	Heart Rate (per min)	Type/Units	Pre	Post
After:		Time:		(diastolic):				

Fasting Blood Sugar:
_____

Water Intake:
total ounces _____

Fitness Log:

Activity	Min

Sleep Log:
Total Hours _____

Notes:
_____
_____
_____
_____
_____
_____
_____
_____
_____
_____

DAILY LOG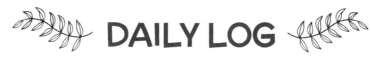

Date: ___/___/_____   **M T W Th F Sa Su**

	Meal	Calories	Fat (g)	Carbs (g)	Sugar (g)	Fiber (g)	Net Carb (carbs-fiber)	Protein (g)	Sodium (mg)
Breakfast									
	Totals:								

Blood Glucose Levels				Blood Pressure Levels			Insulin/Medications		
Before:		Time:		(systolic):		Heart Rate (per min)	Type/Units	Pre	Post
After:		Time:		(diastolic):					

	Meal	Calories	Fat (g)	Carbs (g)	Sugar (g)	Fiber (g)	Net Carb (carbs-fiber)	Protein (g)	Sodium (mg)
Snack #1									
	Totals:								

Blood Glucose Levels				Blood Pressure Levels			Insulin/Medications		
Before:		Time:		(systolic):		Heart Rate (per min)	Type/Units	Pre	Post
After:		Time:		(diastolic):					

	Meal	Calories	Fat (g)	Carbs (g)	Sugar (g)	Fiber (g)	Net Carb (carbs-fiber)	Protein (g)	Sodium (mg)
Lunch									
	Totals:								

Blood Glucose Levels				Blood Pressure Levels			Insulin/Medications		
Before:		Time:		(systolic):		Heart Rate (per min)	Type/Units	Pre	Post
After:		Time:		(diastolic):					

	Meal	Calories	Fat (g)	Carbs (g)	Sugar (g)	Fiber (g)	Net Carb (carbs-fiber)	Protein (g)	Sodium (mg)
Snack #2									
	Totals:								

Blood Glucose Levels				Blood Pressure Levels			Insulin/Medications		
Before:		Time:		(systolic):		Heart Rate (per min)	Type/Units	Pre	Post
After:		Time:		(diastolic):					

	Meal	Calories	Fat (g)	Carbs (g)	Sugar (g)	Fiber (g)	Net Carb (carbs-fiber)	Protein (g)	Sodium (mg)
Dinner									
	Totals:								

Blood Glucose Levels				Blood Pressure Levels			Insulin/Medications		
Before:		Time:		(systolic):		Heart Rate (per min)	Type/Units	Pre	Post
After:		Time:		(diastolic):					

Fasting Blood Sugar:
_____

Water Intake:
total ounces _____

Fitness Log:

Activity	Min

Sleep Log:
Total Hours _____

Notes:
_____
_____
_____
_____
_____
_____
_____

DAILY LOG

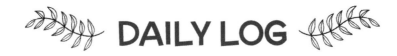

Date: ___/___/_____

M T W Th F Sa Su

Breakfast

	Meal	Calories	Fat (g)	Carbs (g)	Sugar (g)	Fiber (g)	Net Carb (carbs-fiber)	Protein (g)	Sodium (mg)
	Totals:								

Blood Glucose Levels				Blood Pressure Levels			Insulin/Medications		
Before:		Time:		(systolic):		Heart Rate (per min)	Type/Units	Pre	Post
After:		Time:		(diastolic):					

Snack #1

	Totals:								

Blood Glucose Levels				Blood Pressure Levels			Insulin/Medications		
Before:		Time:		(systolic):		Heart Rate (per min)	Type/Units	Pre	Post
After:		Time:		(diastolic):					

Lunch

	Totals:								

Blood Glucose Levels				Blood Pressure Levels			Insulin/Medications		
Before:		Time:		(systolic):		Heart Rate (per min)	Type/Units	Pre	Post
After:		Time:		(diastolic):					

Snack #2

	Totals:								

Blood Glucose Levels				Blood Pressure Levels			Insulin/Medications		
Before:		Time:		(systolic):		Heart Rate (per min)	Type/Units	Pre	Post
After:		Time:		(diastolic):					

Dinner

	Totals:								

Blood Glucose Levels				Blood Pressure Levels			Insulin/Medications		
Before:		Time:		(systolic):		Heart Rate (per min)	Type/Units	Pre	Post
After:		Time:		(diastolic):					

Fasting Blood Sugar:

_____

Water Intake:

total ounces _____

Fitness Log:

Activity	Min

Sleep Log:

Total Hours _____

Notes:

_____
_____
_____
_____
_____
_____
_____
_____
_____

DAILY LOG

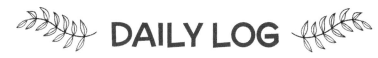

Date: ___/___/_____   **M T W Th F Sa Su**

Breakfast

	Meal	Calories	Fat (g)	Carbs (g)	Sugar (g)	Fiber (g)	Net Carb (carbs-fiber)	Protein (g)	Sodium (mg)
	Totals:								

Blood Glucose Levels			Blood Pressure Levels		Insulin/Medications		
Before:		Time:	(systolic):	Heart Rate (per min)	Type/Units	Pre	Post
After:		Time:	(diastolic):				

Snack #1

	Totals:								

Blood Glucose Levels			Blood Pressure Levels		Insulin/Medications		
Before:		Time:	(systolic):	Heart Rate (per min)	Type/Units	Pre	Post
After:		Time:	(diastolic):				

Lunch

	Totals:								

Blood Glucose Levels			Blood Pressure Levels		Insulin/Medications		
Before:		Time:	(systolic):	Heart Rate (per min)	Type/Units	Pre	Post
After:		Time:	(diastolic):				

Snack #2

	Totals:								

Blood Glucose Levels			Blood Pressure Levels		Insulin/Medications		
Before:		Time:	(systolic):	Heart Rate (per min)	Type/Units	Pre	Post
After:		Time:	(diastolic):				

Dinner

	Totals:								

Blood Glucose Levels			Blood Pressure Levels		Insulin/Medications		
Before:		Time:	(systolic):	Heart Rate (per min)	Type/Units	Pre	Post
After:		Time:	(diastolic):				

Fasting Blood Sugar:

_____

Water Intake:

🍼 🍼 🍼 🍼 🍼 🍼 🍼 🍼

total ounces _____

Fitness Log:

Activity	Min

Sleep Log:

Total Hours _____

Notes:

_____
_____
_____
_____
_____
_____
_____
_____
_____
_____

DAILY LOG

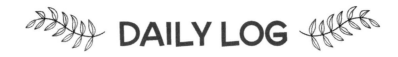

Date: ___/___/_____   **M T W Th F Sa Su**

Breakfast

	Meal	Calories	Fat (g)	Carbs (g)	Sugar (g)	Fiber (g)	Net Carb (carbs-fiber)	Protein (g)	Sodium (mg)
	Totals:								

Blood Glucose Levels				Blood Pressure Levels			Insulin/Medications		
Before:		Time:		(systolic):		Heart Rate (per min)	Type/Units	Pre	Post
After:		Time:		(diastolic):					

Snack #1

	Totals:								

Blood Glucose Levels				Blood Pressure Levels			Insulin/Medications		
Before:		Time:		(systolic):		Heart Rate (per min)	Type/Units	Pre	Post
After:		Time:		(diastolic):					

Lunch

	Totals:								

Blood Glucose Levels				Blood Pressure Levels			Insulin/Medications		
Before:		Time:		(systolic):		Heart Rate (per min)	Type/Units	Pre	Post
After:		Time:		(diastolic):					

Snack #2

	Totals:								

Blood Glucose Levels				Blood Pressure Levels			Insulin/Medications		
Before:		Time:		(systolic):		Heart Rate (per min)	Type/Units	Pre	Post
After:		Time:		(diastolic):					

Dinner

	Totals:								

Blood Glucose Levels				Blood Pressure Levels			Insulin/Medications		
Before:		Time:		(systolic):		Heart Rate (per min)	Type/Units	Pre	Post
After:		Time:		(diastolic):					

Fasting Blood Sugar:

_____

Water Intake:

total ounces _____

Fitness Log:

Activity	Min

Sleep Log:

Total Hours _____

Notes:

_____
_____
_____
_____
_____
_____
_____
_____

DAILY LOG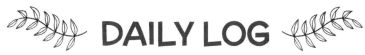

Date: ___/___/_____   **M T W Th F Sa Su**

Breakfast

Meal	Calories	Fat (g)	Carbs (g)	Sugar (g)	Fiber (g)	Net Carb (carbs-fiber)	Protein (g)	Sodium (mg)
Totals:								

Blood Glucose Levels		Blood Pressure Levels		Insulin/Medications		
Before:	Time:	(systolic):	Heart Rate (per min)	Type/Units	Pre	Post
After:	Time:	(diastolic):				

Snack #1

Meal	Calories	Fat (g)	Carbs (g)	Sugar (g)	Fiber (g)	Net Carb (carbs-fiber)	Protein (g)	Sodium (mg)
Totals:								

Blood Glucose Levels		Blood Pressure Levels		Insulin/Medications		
Before:	Time:	(systolic):	Heart Rate (per min)	Type/Units	Pre	Post
After:	Time:	(diastolic):				

Lunch

Meal	Calories	Fat (g)	Carbs (g)	Sugar (g)	Fiber (g)	Net Carb (carbs-fiber)	Protein (g)	Sodium (mg)
Totals:								

Blood Glucose Levels		Blood Pressure Levels		Insulin/Medications		
Before:	Time:	(systolic):	Heart Rate (per min)	Type/Units	Pre	Post
After:	Time:	(diastolic):				

Snack #2

Meal	Calories	Fat (g)	Carbs (g)	Sugar (g)	Fiber (g)	Net Carb (carbs-fiber)	Protein (g)	Sodium (mg)
Totals:								

Blood Glucose Levels		Blood Pressure Levels		Insulin/Medications		
Before:	Time:	(systolic):	Heart Rate (per min)	Type/Units	Pre	Post
After:	Time:	(diastolic):				

Dinner

Meal	Calories	Fat (g)	Carbs (g)	Sugar (g)	Fiber (g)	Net Carb (carbs-fiber)	Protein (g)	Sodium (mg)
Totals:								

Blood Glucose Levels		Blood Pressure Levels		Insulin/Medications		
Before:	Time:	(systolic):	Heart Rate (per min)	Type/Units	Pre	Post
After:	Time:	(diastolic):				

Fasting Blood Sugar:

_____

Water Intake:

total ounces _____

Fitness Log:

Activity	Min

Sleep Log:

Total Hours _____

Notes:

_____
_____
_____
_____
_____
_____
_____
_____

DAILY LOG

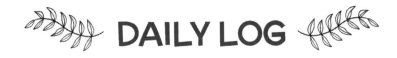

Date: ___/___/_____   **M T W Th F Sa Su**

Breakfast

	Meal	Calories	Fat (g)	Carbs (g)	Sugar (g)	Fiber (g)	Net Carb (carbs-fiber)	Protein (g)	Sodium (mg)
Totals:									

Blood Glucose Levels				Blood Pressure Levels			Insulin/Medications		
						Heart Rate (per min)	Type/Units	Pre	Post
Before:		Time:		(systolic):					
After:		Time:		(diastolic):					

Snack #1

Totals:									

Blood Glucose Levels				Blood Pressure Levels			Insulin/Medications		
						Heart Rate (per min)	Type/Units	Pre	Post
Before:		Time:		(systolic):					
After:		Time:		(diastolic):					

Lunch

Totals:									

Blood Glucose Levels				Blood Pressure Levels			Insulin/Medications		
						Heart Rate (per min)	Type/Units	Pre	Post
Before:		Time:		(systolic):					
After:		Time:		(diastolic):					

Snack #2

Totals:									

Blood Glucose Levels				Blood Pressure Levels			Insulin/Medications		
						Heart Rate (per min)	Type/Units	Pre	Post
Before:		Time:		(systolic):					
After:		Time:		(diastolic):					

Dinner

Totals:									

Blood Glucose Levels				Blood Pressure Levels			Insulin/Medications		
						Heart Rate (per min)	Type/Units	Pre	Post
Before:		Time:		(systolic):					
After:		Time:		(diastolic):					

Fasting Blood Sugar:
_____

Water Intake:
total ounces _____

Fitness Log:
Activity	Min

Sleep Log:
Total Hours _____

Notes:
_____
_____
_____
_____
_____
_____
_____
_____

DAILY LOG

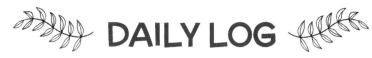

Date: ____/____/_____   **M T W Th F Sa Su**

Breakfast

Meal	Calories	Fat (g)	Carbs (g)	Sugar (g)	Fiber (g)	Net Carb (carbs-fiber)	Protein (g)	Sodium (mg)
Totals:								

Blood Glucose Levels		Blood Pressure Levels		Insulin/Medications		
Before:	Time:	(systolic):	Heart Rate (per min)	Type/Units	Pre	Post
After:	Time:	(diastolic):				

Snack #1

Totals:								

Blood Glucose Levels		Blood Pressure Levels		Insulin/Medications		
Before:	Time:	(systolic):	Heart Rate (per min)	Type/Units	Pre	Post
After:	Time:	(diastolic):				

Lunch

Totals:								

Blood Glucose Levels		Blood Pressure Levels		Insulin/Medications		
Before:	Time:	(systolic):	Heart Rate (per min)	Type/Units	Pre	Post
After:	Time:	(diastolic):				

Snack #2

Totals:								

Blood Glucose Levels		Blood Pressure Levels		Insulin/Medications		
Before:	Time:	(systolic):	Heart Rate (per min)	Type/Units	Pre	Post
After:	Time:	(diastolic):				

Dinner

Totals:								

Blood Glucose Levels		Blood Pressure Levels		Insulin/Medications		
Before:	Time:	(systolic):	Heart Rate (per min)	Type/Units	Pre	Post
After:	Time:	(diastolic):				

Fasting Blood Sugar:

_____

Water Intake:

total ounces _____

Fitness Log:

Activity	Min

Sleep Log:

Total Hours _____

Notes:

_____
_____
_____
_____
_____
_____
_____
_____
_____
_____

DAILY LOG

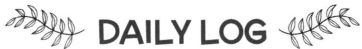

Date: ___/___/_____   **M T W Th F Sa Su**

Breakfast

Meal		Calories	Fat (g)	Carbs (g)	Sugar (g)	Fiber (g)	Net Carb (carbs-fiber)	Protein (g)	Sodium (mg)
	Totals:								

Blood Glucose Levels			Blood Pressure Levels			Insulin/Medications		
Before:		Time:	(systolic):		Heart Rate (per min)	Type/Units	Pre	Post
After:		Time:	(diastolic):					

Snack #1

	Totals:								

Blood Glucose Levels			Blood Pressure Levels			Insulin/Medications		
Before:		Time:	(systolic):		Heart Rate (per min)	Type/Units	Pre	Post
After:		Time:	(diastolic):					

Lunch

	Totals:								

Blood Glucose Levels			Blood Pressure Levels			Insulin/Medications		
Before:		Time:	(systolic):		Heart Rate (per min)	Type/Units	Pre	Post
After:		Time:	(diastolic):					

Snack #2

	Totals:								

Blood Glucose Levels			Blood Pressure Levels			Insulin/Medications		
Before:		Time:	(systolic):		Heart Rate (per min)	Type/Units	Pre	Post
After:		Time:	(diastolic):					

Dinner

	Totals:								

Blood Glucose Levels			Blood Pressure Levels			Insulin/Medications		
Before:		Time:	(systolic):		Heart Rate (per min)	Type/Units	Pre	Post
After:		Time:	(diastolic):					

Fasting Blood Sugar:

_____

Water Intake:

🍼🍼🍼🍼🍼🍼🍼🍼

total ounces _____

Fitness Log:

Activity	Min

Sleep Log:

Total Hours _____

Notes:

_____
_____
_____
_____
_____
_____
_____
_____
_____
_____

DAILY LOG

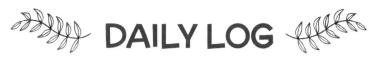

Date: ___/___/_____   **M T W Th F Sa Su**

Breakfast

Meal	Calories	Fat (g)	Carbs (g)	Sugar (g)	Fiber (g)	Net Carb (carbs-fiber)	Protein (g)	Sodium (mg)
Totals:								

Blood Glucose Levels			Blood Pressure Levels			Insulin/Medications		
Before:		Time:	(systolic):		Heart Rate (per min)	Type/Units	Pre	Post
After:		Time:	(diastolic):					

Fasting Blood Sugar:
_____

Snack #1

Totals:								

Blood Glucose Levels			Blood Pressure Levels			Insulin/Medications		
Before:		Time:	(systolic):		Heart Rate (per min)	Type/Units	Pre	Post
After:		Time:	(diastolic):					

Water Intake:
total ounces _____

Lunch

Totals:								

Blood Glucose Levels			Blood Pressure Levels			Insulin/Medications		
Before:		Time:	(systolic):		Heart Rate (per min)	Type/Units	Pre	Post
After:		Time:	(diastolic):					

Fitness Log:
Activity	Min

Sleep Log:
Total Hours _____

Snack #2

Totals:								

Blood Glucose Levels			Blood Pressure Levels			Insulin/Medications		
Before:		Time:	(systolic):		Heart Rate (per min)	Type/Units	Pre	Post
After:		Time:	(diastolic):					

Notes:
_____
_____

Dinner

Totals:								

Blood Glucose Levels			Blood Pressure Levels			Insulin/Medications		
Before:		Time:	(systolic):		Heart Rate (per min)	Type/Units	Pre	Post
After:		Time:	(diastolic):					

DAILY LOG

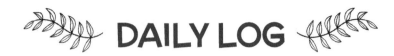

Date: ____/____/_____   **M T W Th F Sa Su**

Breakfast

Meal	Calories	Fat (g)	Carbs (g)	Sugar (g)	Fiber (g)	Net Carb (carbs-fiber)	Protein (g)	Sodium (mg)
Totals:								

Blood Glucose Levels		Blood Pressure Levels	Heart Rate (per min)	Insulin/Medications		
Before:	Time:	(systolic):		Type/Units	Pre	Post
After:	Time:	(diastolic):				

Snack #1

Totals:								

Blood Glucose Levels		Blood Pressure Levels	Heart Rate (per min)	Insulin/Medications		
Before:	Time:	(systolic):		Type/Units	Pre	Post
After:	Time:	(diastolic):				

Lunch

Totals:								

Blood Glucose Levels		Blood Pressure Levels	Heart Rate (per min)	Insulin/Medications		
Before:	Time:	(systolic):		Type/Units	Pre	Post
After:	Time:	(diastolic):				

Snack #2

Totals:								

Blood Glucose Levels		Blood Pressure Levels	Heart Rate (per min)	Insulin/Medications		
Before:	Time:	(systolic):		Type/Units	Pre	Post
After:	Time:	(diastolic):				

Dinner

Totals:								

Blood Glucose Levels		Blood Pressure Levels	Heart Rate (per min)	Insulin/Medications		
Before:	Time:	(systolic):		Type/Units	Pre	Post
After:	Time:	(diastolic):				

Fasting Blood Sugar:
_____

Water Intake:
total ounces _____

Fitness Log:

Activity	Min

Sleep Log:
Total Hours _____

Notes:

DAILY LOG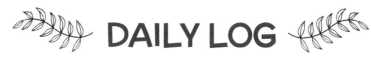

Date: ____/____/_____   M T W Th F Sa Su

Breakfast

Meal	Calories	Fat (g)	Carbs (g)	Sugar (g)	Fiber (g)	Net Carb (carbs-fiber)	Protein (g)	Sodium (mg)
Totals:								

Blood Glucose Levels			Blood Pressure Levels			Insulin/Medications		
Before:		Time:	(systolic):		Heart Rate (per min)	Type/Units	Pre	Post
After:		Time:	(diastolic):					

Snack #1

Totals:								

Blood Glucose Levels			Blood Pressure Levels			Insulin/Medications		
Before:		Time:	(systolic):		Heart Rate (per min)	Type/Units	Pre	Post
After:		Time:	(diastolic):					

Lunch

Totals:								

Blood Glucose Levels			Blood Pressure Levels			Insulin/Medications		
Before:		Time:	(systolic):		Heart Rate (per min)	Type/Units	Pre	Post
After:		Time:	(diastolic):					

Snack #2

Totals:								

Blood Glucose Levels			Blood Pressure Levels			Insulin/Medications		
Before:		Time:	(systolic):		Heart Rate (per min)	Type/Units	Pre	Post
After:		Time:	(diastolic):					

Dinner

Totals:								

Blood Glucose Levels			Blood Pressure Levels			Insulin/Medications		
Before:		Time:	(systolic):		Heart Rate (per min)	Type/Units	Pre	Post
After:		Time:	(diastolic):					

Fasting Blood Sugar:
_____

Water Intake:
total ounces _____

Fitness Log:

Activity	Min

Sleep Log:
Total Hours _____

Notes:
_____
_____
_____
_____
_____
_____
_____
_____
_____

DAILY LOG

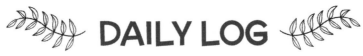

Date: ___/___/_____   **M T W Th F Sa Su**

Breakfast

	Meal	Calories	Fat (g)	Carbs (g)	Sugar (g)	Fiber (g)	Net Carb (carbs-fiber)	Protein (g)	Sodium (mg)
	Totals:								

Blood Glucose Levels				Blood Pressure Levels			Insulin/Medications		
Before:		Time:		(systolic):		Heart Rate (per min)	Type/Units	Pre	Post
After:		Time:		(diastolic):					

Snack #1

	Totals:								

Blood Glucose Levels				Blood Pressure Levels			Insulin/Medications		
Before:		Time:		(systolic):		Heart Rate (per min)	Type/Units	Pre	Post
After:		Time:		(diastolic):					

Lunch

	Totals:								

Blood Glucose Levels				Blood Pressure Levels			Insulin/Medications		
Before:		Time:		(systolic):		Heart Rate (per min)	Type/Units	Pre	Post
After:		Time:		(diastolic):					

Snack #2

	Totals:								

Blood Glucose Levels				Blood Pressure Levels			Insulin/Medications		
Before:		Time:		(systolic):		Heart Rate (per min)	Type/Units	Pre	Post
After:		Time:		(diastolic):					

Dinner

	Totals:								

Blood Glucose Levels				Blood Pressure Levels			Insulin/Medications		
Before:		Time:		(systolic):		Heart Rate (per min)	Type/Units	Pre	Post
After:		Time:		(diastolic):					

Fasting Blood Sugar:

_____

Water Intake:

total ounces _____

Fitness Log:

Activity	Min

Sleep Log:

Total Hours _____

Notes:

_____
_____
_____
_____
_____
_____
_____
_____
_____
_____
_____

DAILY LOG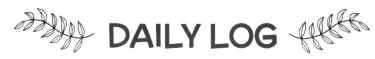

Date: ___/___/_____   **M T W Th F Sa Su**

Breakfast

Meal	Calories	Fat (g)	Carbs (g)	Sugar (g)	Fiber (g)	Net Carb (carbs-fiber)	Protein (g)	Sodium (mg)
Totals:								

Blood Glucose Levels			Blood Pressure Levels			Insulin/Medications		
Before:		Time:	(systolic):		Heart Rate (per min)	Type/Units	Pre	Post
After:		Time:	(diastolic):					

Snack #1

Meal	Calories	Fat (g)	Carbs (g)	Sugar (g)	Fiber (g)	Net Carb (carbs-fiber)	Protein (g)	Sodium (mg)
Totals:								

Blood Glucose Levels			Blood Pressure Levels			Insulin/Medications		
Before:		Time:	(systolic):		Heart Rate (per min)	Type/Units	Pre	Post
After:		Time:	(diastolic):					

Lunch

Meal	Calories	Fat (g)	Carbs (g)	Sugar (g)	Fiber (g)	Net Carb (carbs-fiber)	Protein (g)	Sodium (mg)
Totals:								

Blood Glucose Levels			Blood Pressure Levels			Insulin/Medications		
Before:		Time:	(systolic):		Heart Rate (per min)	Type/Units	Pre	Post
After:		Time:	(diastolic):					

Snack #2

Meal	Calories	Fat (g)	Carbs (g)	Sugar (g)	Fiber (g)	Net Carb (carbs-fiber)	Protein (g)	Sodium (mg)
Totals:								

Blood Glucose Levels			Blood Pressure Levels			Insulin/Medications		
Before:		Time:	(systolic):		Heart Rate (per min)	Type/Units	Pre	Post
After:		Time:	(diastolic):					

Dinner

Meal	Calories	Fat (g)	Carbs (g)	Sugar (g)	Fiber (g)	Net Carb (carbs-fiber)	Protein (g)	Sodium (mg)
Totals:								

Blood Glucose Levels			Blood Pressure Levels			Insulin/Medications		
Before:		Time:	(systolic):		Heart Rate (per min)	Type/Units	Pre	Post
After:		Time:	(diastolic):					

Fasting Blood Sugar:

_____

Water Intake:

total ounces _____

Fitness Log:

Activity	Min

Sleep Log:

Total Hours _____

Notes:

_____
_____
_____
_____
_____
_____
_____
_____
_____
_____

DAILY LOG

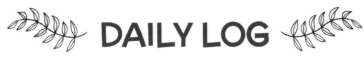

Date: ___/___/_____   **M T W Th F Sa Su**

Breakfast

	Meal	Calories	Fat (g)	Carbs (g)	Sugar (g)	Fiber (g)	Net Carb (carbs-fiber)	Protein (g)	Sodium (mg)
	Totals:								

Blood Glucose Levels				Blood Pressure Levels		Insulin/Medications		
Before:		Time:		(systolic):	Heart Rate (per min)	Type/Units	Pre	Post
After:		Time:		(diastolic):				

Snack #1

	Totals:								

Blood Glucose Levels				Blood Pressure Levels		Insulin/Medications		
Before:		Time:		(systolic):	Heart Rate (per min)	Type/Units	Pre	Post
After:		Time:		(diastolic):				

Lunch

	Totals:								

Blood Glucose Levels				Blood Pressure Levels		Insulin/Medications		
Before:		Time:		(systolic):	Heart Rate (per min)	Type/Units	Pre	Post
After:		Time:		(diastolic):				

Snack #2

	Totals:								

Blood Glucose Levels				Blood Pressure Levels		Insulin/Medications		
Before:		Time:		(systolic):	Heart Rate (per min)	Type/Units	Pre	Post
After:		Time:		(diastolic):				

Dinner

	Totals:								

Blood Glucose Levels				Blood Pressure Levels		Insulin/Medications		
Before:		Time:		(systolic):	Heart Rate (per min)	Type/Units	Pre	Post
After:		Time:		(diastolic):				

Fasting Blood Sugar:

_____

Water Intake:

total ounces _____

Fitness Log:

Activity   Min

Sleep Log:

Total Hours _____

Notes:

DAILY LOG

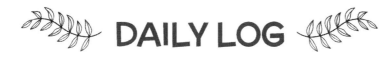

Date: ____/____/_____   **M T W Th F Sa Su**

Breakfast

	Meal	Calories	Fat (g)	Carbs (g)	Sugar (g)	Fiber (g)	Net Carb (carbs-fiber)	Protein (g)	Sodium (mg)
	Totals:								

Blood Glucose Levels			Blood Pressure Levels		Insulin/Medications		
Before:		Time:	(systolic):	Heart Rate (per min)	Type/Units	Pre	Post
After:		Time:	(diastolic):				

Snack #1

	Totals:								

Blood Glucose Levels			Blood Pressure Levels		Insulin/Medications		
Before:		Time:	(systolic):	Heart Rate (per min)	Type/Units	Pre	Post
After:		Time:	(diastolic):				

Lunch

	Totals:								

Blood Glucose Levels			Blood Pressure Levels		Insulin/Medications		
Before:		Time:	(systolic):	Heart Rate (per min)	Type/Units	Pre	Post
After:		Time:	(diastolic):				

Snack #2

	Totals:								

Blood Glucose Levels			Blood Pressure Levels		Insulin/Medications		
Before:		Time:	(systolic):	Heart Rate (per min)	Type/Units	Pre	Post
After:		Time:	(diastolic):				

Dinner

	Totals:								

Blood Glucose Levels			Blood Pressure Levels		Insulin/Medications		
Before:		Time:	(systolic):	Heart Rate (per min)	Type/Units	Pre	Post
After:		Time:	(diastolic):				

Fasting Blood Sugar:

_____

Water Intake:

total ounces _____

Fitness Log:

Activity	Min

Sleep Log:

Total Hours _____

Notes:

_____
_____
_____
_____
_____
_____
_____
_____

DAILY LOG

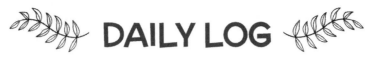

Date: ___/___/_____   **M T W Th F Sa Su**

Breakfast

	Meal	Calories	Fat (g)	Carbs (g)	Sugar (g)	Fiber (g)	Net Carb (carbs-fiber)	Protein (g)	Sodium (mg)
	Totals:								

Blood Glucose Levels			Blood Pressure Levels			Insulin/Medications		
Before:		Time:	(systolic):		Heart Rate (per min)	Type/Units	Pre	Post
After:		Time:	(diastolic):					

Fasting Blood Sugar:

_____

Snack #1

	Totals:								

Blood Glucose Levels			Blood Pressure Levels			Insulin/Medications		
Before:		Time:	(systolic):		Heart Rate (per min)	Type/Units	Pre	Post
After:		Time:	(diastolic):					

Water Intake:

🍶🍶🍶🍶🍶🍶🍶🍶

total ounces _____

Fitness Log:

Activity   Min

Lunch

	Totals:								

Blood Glucose Levels			Blood Pressure Levels			Insulin/Medications		
Before:		Time:	(systolic):		Heart Rate (per min)	Type/Units	Pre	Post
After:		Time:	(diastolic):					

Sleep Log:

Total Hours _____

Snack #2

	Totals:								

Blood Glucose Levels			Blood Pressure Levels			Insulin/Medications		
Before:		Time:	(systolic):		Heart Rate (per min)	Type/Units	Pre	Post
After:		Time:	(diastolic):					

Notes:

Dinner

	Totals:								

Blood Glucose Levels			Blood Pressure Levels			Insulin/Medications		
Before:		Time:	(systolic):		Heart Rate (per min)	Type/Units	Pre	Post
After:		Time:	(diastolic):					

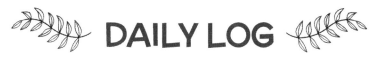

DAILY LOG

Date: ___/___/_____   **M T W Th F Sa Su**

Breakfast

Meal	Calories	Fat (g)	Carbs (g)	Sugar (g)	Fiber (g)	Net Carb (carbs-fiber)	Protein (g)	Sodium (mg)
Totals:								

Blood Glucose Levels		Blood Pressure Levels		Insulin/Medications		
Before:	Time:	(systolic):	Heart Rate (per min)	Type/Units	Pre	Post
After:	Time:	(diastolic):				

Snack #1

Totals:								

Blood Glucose Levels		Blood Pressure Levels		Insulin/Medications		
Before:	Time:	(systolic):	Heart Rate (per min)	Type/Units	Pre	Post
After:	Time:	(diastolic):				

Lunch

Totals:								

Blood Glucose Levels		Blood Pressure Levels		Insulin/Medications		
Before:	Time:	(systolic):	Heart Rate (per min)	Type/Units	Pre	Post
After:	Time:	(diastolic):				

Snack #2

Totals:								

Blood Glucose Levels		Blood Pressure Levels		Insulin/Medications		
Before:	Time:	(systolic):	Heart Rate (per min)	Type/Units	Pre	Post
After:	Time:	(diastolic):				

Dinner

Totals:								

Blood Glucose Levels		Blood Pressure Levels		Insulin/Medications		
Before:	Time:	(systolic):	Heart Rate (per min)	Type/Units	Pre	Post
After:	Time:	(diastolic):				

Fasting Blood Sugar:

_____

Water Intake:

total ounces _____

Fitness Log:

Activity	Min

Sleep Log:

Total Hours _____

Notes:

_____
_____
_____
_____
_____
_____
_____
_____

DAILY LOG

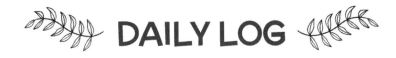

Date: ___/___/_____   M T W Th F Sa Su

Breakfast

	Meal	Calories	Fat (g)	Carbs (g)	Sugar (g)	Fiber (g)	Net Carb (carbs-fiber)	Protein (g)	Sodium (mg)
	Totals:								

Blood Glucose Levels				Blood Pressure Levels		Insulin/Medications		
Before:		Time:		(systolic):	Heart Rate (per min)	Type/Units	Pre	Post
After:		Time:		(diastolic):				

Snack #1

	Totals:								

Blood Glucose Levels				Blood Pressure Levels		Insulin/Medications		
Before:		Time:		(systolic):	Heart Rate (per min)	Type/Units	Pre	Post
After:		Time:		(diastolic):				

Lunch

	Totals:								

Blood Glucose Levels				Blood Pressure Levels		Insulin/Medications		
Before:		Time:		(systolic):	Heart Rate (per min)	Type/Units	Pre	Post
After:		Time:		(diastolic):				

Snack #2

	Totals:								

Blood Glucose Levels				Blood Pressure Levels		Insulin/Medications		
Before:		Time:		(systolic):	Heart Rate (per min)	Type/Units	Pre	Post
After:		Time:		(diastolic):				

Dinner

	Totals:								

Blood Glucose Levels				Blood Pressure Levels		Insulin/Medications		
Before:		Time:		(systolic):	Heart Rate (per min)	Type/Units	Pre	Post
After:		Time:		(diastolic):				

Fasting Blood Sugar:

_____

Water Intake:

total ounces _____

Fitness Log:

Activity	Min

Sleep Log:

Total Hours _____

Notes:

_____
_____
_____
_____
_____
_____
_____
_____
_____
_____
_____

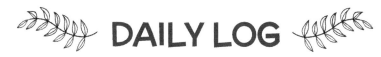

DAILY LOG

Date: ___/___/_____   **M T W Th F Sa Su**

Breakfast

Meal	Calories	Fat (g)	Carbs (g)	Sugar (g)	Fiber (g)	Net Carb (carbs-fiber)	Protein (g)	Sodium (mg)
Totals:								

Blood Glucose Levels			Blood Pressure Levels			Insulin/Medications		
					Heart Rate (per min)	Type/Units	Pre	Post
Before:		Time:	(systolic):					
After:		Time:	(diastolic):					

Snack #1

Totals:								

Blood Glucose Levels			Blood Pressure Levels			Insulin/Medications		
					Heart Rate (per min)	Type/Units	Pre	Post
Before:		Time:	(systolic):					
After:		Time:	(diastolic):					

Lunch

Totals:								

Blood Glucose Levels			Blood Pressure Levels			Insulin/Medications		
					Heart Rate (per min)	Type/Units	Pre	Post
Before:		Time:	(systolic):					
After:		Time:	(diastolic):					

Snack #2

Totals:								

Blood Glucose Levels			Blood Pressure Levels			Insulin/Medications		
					Heart Rate (per min)	Type/Units	Pre	Post
Before:		Time:	(systolic):					
After:		Time:	(diastolic):					

Dinner

Totals:								

Blood Glucose Levels			Blood Pressure Levels			Insulin/Medications		
					Heart Rate (per min)	Type/Units	Pre	Post
Before:		Time:	(systolic):					
After:		Time:	(diastolic):					

Fasting Blood Sugar:

_____

Water Intake:

total ounces _____

Fitness Log:

Activity	Min

Sleep Log:

Total Hours _____

Notes:

_____
_____
_____
_____
_____
_____
_____
_____
_____
_____
_____
_____
_____

DAILY LOG

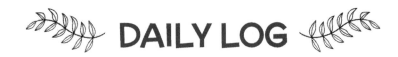

Date: ___/___/_____

M T W Th F Sa Su

Breakfast

	Meal	Calories	Fat (g)	Carbs (g)	Sugar (g)	Fiber (g)	Net Carb (carbs-fiber)	Protein (g)	Sodium (mg)
	Totals:								

Blood Glucose Levels				Blood Pressure Levels		Insulin/Medications		
Before:		Time:		(systolic):	Heart Rate (per min)	Type/Units	Pre	Post
After:		Time:		(diastolic):				

Snack #1

	Totals:								

Blood Glucose Levels				Blood Pressure Levels		Insulin/Medications		
Before:		Time:		(systolic):	Heart Rate (per min)	Type/Units	Pre	Post
After:		Time:		(diastolic):				

Lunch

	Totals:								

Blood Glucose Levels				Blood Pressure Levels		Insulin/Medications		
Before:		Time:		(systolic):	Heart Rate (per min)	Type/Units	Pre	Post
After:		Time:		(diastolic):				

Snack #2

	Totals:								

Blood Glucose Levels				Blood Pressure Levels		Insulin/Medications		
Before:		Time:		(systolic):	Heart Rate (per min)	Type/Units	Pre	Post
After:		Time:		(diastolic):				

Dinner

	Totals:								

Blood Glucose Levels				Blood Pressure Levels		Insulin/Medications		
Before:		Time:		(systolic):	Heart Rate (per min)	Type/Units	Pre	Post
After:		Time:		(diastolic):				

Fasting Blood Sugar:
_____

Water Intake:
total ounces _____

Fitness Log:

Activity	Min

Sleep Log:
Total Hours _____

Notes:

DAILY LOG

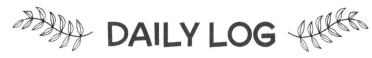

Date: ___/___/_____

M T W Th F Sa Su

Breakfast

Meal	Calories	Fat (g)	Carbs (g)	Sugar (g)	Fiber (g)	Net Carb (carbs-fiber)	Protein (g)	Sodium (mg)
Totals:								

Blood Glucose Levels			Blood Pressure Levels			Insulin/Medications		
Before:		Time:	(systolic):		Heart Rate (per min)	Type/Units	Pre	Post
After:		Time:	(diastolic):					

Snack #1

Totals:								

Blood Glucose Levels			Blood Pressure Levels			Insulin/Medications		
Before:		Time:	(systolic):		Heart Rate (per min)	Type/Units	Pre	Post
After:		Time:	(diastolic):					

Lunch

Totals:								

Blood Glucose Levels			Blood Pressure Levels			Insulin/Medications		
Before:		Time:	(systolic):		Heart Rate (per min)	Type/Units	Pre	Post
After:		Time:	(diastolic):					

Snack #2

Totals:								

Blood Glucose Levels			Blood Pressure Levels			Insulin/Medications		
Before:		Time:	(systolic):		Heart Rate (per min)	Type/Units	Pre	Post
After:		Time:	(diastolic):					

Dinner

Totals:								

Blood Glucose Levels			Blood Pressure Levels			Insulin/Medications		
Before:		Time:	(systolic):		Heart Rate (per min)	Type/Units	Pre	Post
After:		Time:	(diastolic):					

Fasting Blood Sugar:

_____

Water Intake:

total ounces _____

Fitness Log:

Activity	Min

Sleep Log:

Total Hours _____

Notes:

DAILY LOG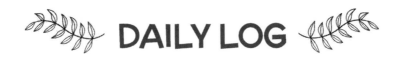

Date: ___/___/_____   **M T W Th F Sa Su**

Breakfast

	Meal	Calories	Fat (g)	Carbs (g)	Sugar (g)	Fiber (g)	Net Carb (carbs-fiber)	Protein (g)	Sodium (mg)
	Totals:								

Blood Glucose Levels				Blood Pressure Levels			Insulin/Medications		
Before:		Time:		(systolic):		Heart Rate (per min)	Type/Units	Pre	Post
After:		Time:		(diastolic):					

Fasting Blood Sugar:

_____

Snack #1

	Totals:								

Blood Glucose Levels				Blood Pressure Levels			Insulin/Medications		
Before:		Time:		(systolic):		Heart Rate (per min)	Type/Units	Pre	Post
After:		Time:		(diastolic):					

Water Intake:

🍶🍶🍶🍶🍶🍶🍶🍶

total ounces _____

Fitness Log:

Activity	Min

Lunch

	Totals:								

Blood Glucose Levels				Blood Pressure Levels			Insulin/Medications		
Before:		Time:		(systolic):		Heart Rate (per min)	Type/Units	Pre	Post
After:		Time:		(diastolic):					

Sleep Log:

Total Hours _____

Snack #2

	Totals:								

Blood Glucose Levels				Blood Pressure Levels			Insulin/Medications		
Before:		Time:		(systolic):		Heart Rate (per min)	Type/Units	Pre	Post
After:		Time:		(diastolic):					

Notes:

_____
_____
_____
_____

Dinner

	Totals:								

Blood Glucose Levels				Blood Pressure Levels			Insulin/Medications		
Before:		Time:		(systolic):		Heart Rate (per min)	Type/Units	Pre	Post
After:		Time:		(diastolic):					

DAILY LOG

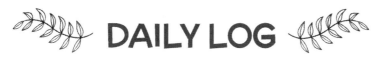

Date: ___/___/_____   **M T W Th F Sa Su**

Breakfast

	Meal	Calories	Fat (g)	Carbs (g)	Sugar (g)	Fiber (g)	Net Carb (carbs-fiber)	Protein (g)	Sodium (mg)
	Totals:								

Blood Glucose Levels			Blood Pressure Levels		Insulin/Medications		
Before:		Time:	(systolic):	Heart Rate (per min)	Type/Units	Pre	Post
After:		Time:	(diastolic):				

Snack #1

	Totals:								

Blood Glucose Levels			Blood Pressure Levels		Insulin/Medications		
Before:		Time:	(systolic):	Heart Rate (per min)	Type/Units	Pre	Post
After:		Time:	(diastolic):				

Lunch

	Totals:								

Blood Glucose Levels			Blood Pressure Levels		Insulin/Medications		
Before:		Time:	(systolic):	Heart Rate (per min)	Type/Units	Pre	Post
After:		Time:	(diastolic):				

Snack #2

	Totals:								

Blood Glucose Levels			Blood Pressure Levels		Insulin/Medications		
Before:		Time:	(systolic):	Heart Rate (per min)	Type/Units	Pre	Post
After:		Time:	(diastolic):				

Dinner

	Totals:								

Blood Glucose Levels			Blood Pressure Levels		Insulin/Medications		
Before:		Time:	(systolic):	Heart Rate (per min)	Type/Units	Pre	Post
After:		Time:	(diastolic):				

Fasting Blood Sugar:

_____

Water Intake:

total ounces _____

Fitness Log:

Activity	Min

Sleep Log:

Total Hours _____

Notes:

_____
_____
_____
_____
_____
_____
_____
_____
_____
_____

DAILY LOG

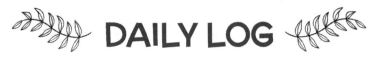

Date: ___/___/_____   M T W Th F Sa Su

Breakfast

Meal	Calories	Fat (g)	Carbs (g)	Sugar (g)	Fiber (g)	Net Carb (carbs-fiber)	Protein (g)	Sodium (mg)
Totals:								

Blood Glucose Levels			Blood Pressure Levels			Insulin/Medications		
Before:		Time:	(systolic):		Heart Rate (per min)	Type/Units	Pre	Post
After:		Time:	(diastolic):					

Snack #1

Totals:								

Blood Glucose Levels			Blood Pressure Levels			Insulin/Medications		
Before:		Time:	(systolic):		Heart Rate (per min)	Type/Units	Pre	Post
After:		Time:	(diastolic):					

Lunch

Totals:								

Blood Glucose Levels			Blood Pressure Levels			Insulin/Medications		
Before:		Time:	(systolic):		Heart Rate (per min)	Type/Units	Pre	Post
After:		Time:	(diastolic):					

Snack #2

Totals:								

Blood Glucose Levels			Blood Pressure Levels			Insulin/Medications		
Before:		Time:	(systolic):		Heart Rate (per min)	Type/Units	Pre	Post
After:		Time:	(diastolic):					

Dinner

Totals:								

Blood Glucose Levels			Blood Pressure Levels			Insulin/Medications		
Before:		Time:	(systolic):		Heart Rate (per min)	Type/Units	Pre	Post
After:		Time:	(diastolic):					

Fasting Blood Sugar:
_____

Water Intake:
total ounces _____

Fitness Log:

Activity	Min

Sleep Log:
Total Hours _____

Notes:
_____
_____
_____
_____
_____
_____
_____
_____
_____
_____
_____

DAILY LOG

Date: ___/___/_____   **M T W Th F Sa Su**

Breakfast

Meal	Calories	Fat (g)	Carbs (g)	Sugar (g)	Fiber (g)	Net Carb (carbs-fiber)	Protein (g)	Sodium (mg)
Totals:								

Blood Glucose Levels				Blood Pressure Levels			Insulin/Medications		
Before:		Time:		(systolic):		Heart Rate (per min)	Type/Units	Pre	Post
After:		Time:		(diastolic):					

Snack #1

Totals:								

Blood Glucose Levels				Blood Pressure Levels			Insulin/Medications		
Before:		Time:		(systolic):		Heart Rate (per min)	Type/Units	Pre	Post
After:		Time:		(diastolic):					

Lunch

Totals:								

Blood Glucose Levels				Blood Pressure Levels			Insulin/Medications		
Before:		Time:		(systolic):		Heart Rate (per min)	Type/Units	Pre	Post
After:		Time:		(diastolic):					

Snack #2

Totals:								

Blood Glucose Levels				Blood Pressure Levels			Insulin/Medications		
Before:		Time:		(systolic):		Heart Rate (per min)	Type/Units	Pre	Post
After:		Time:		(diastolic):					

Dinner

Totals:								

Blood Glucose Levels				Blood Pressure Levels			Insulin/Medications		
Before:		Time:		(systolic):		Heart Rate (per min)	Type/Units	Pre	Post
After:		Time:		(diastolic):					

Fasting Blood Sugar:
_____

Water Intake:
total ounces _____

Fitness Log:

Activity	Min

Sleep Log:
Total Hours _____

Notes:

DAILY LOG

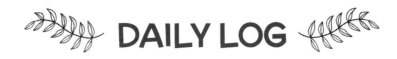

Date: ____/____/_____   M T W Th F Sa Su

Breakfast

Meal	Calories	Fat (g)	Carbs (g)	Sugar (g)	Fiber (g)	Net Carb (carbs-fiber)	Protein (g)	Sodium (mg)
Totals:								

Blood Glucose Levels				Blood Pressure Levels		Insulin/Medications		
Before:		Time:		(systolic):		Type/Units	Pre	Post
After:		Time:		(diastolic):	Heart Rate (per min)			

Snack #1

Totals:								

Blood Glucose Levels				Blood Pressure Levels		Insulin/Medications		
Before:		Time:		(systolic):		Type/Units	Pre	Post
After:		Time:		(diastolic):	Heart Rate (per min)			

Lunch

Totals:								

Blood Glucose Levels				Blood Pressure Levels		Insulin/Medications		
Before:		Time:		(systolic):		Type/Units	Pre	Post
After:		Time:		(diastolic):	Heart Rate (per min)			

Snack #2

Totals:								

Blood Glucose Levels				Blood Pressure Levels		Insulin/Medications		
Before:		Time:		(systolic):		Type/Units	Pre	Post
After:		Time:		(diastolic):	Heart Rate (per min)			

Dinner

Totals:								

Blood Glucose Levels				Blood Pressure Levels		Insulin/Medications		
Before:		Time:		(systolic):		Type/Units	Pre	Post
After:		Time:		(diastolic):	Heart Rate (per min)			

Fasting Blood Sugar:

_____

Water Intake:

total ounces _____

Fitness Log:

Activity   Min

Sleep Log:

Total Hours _____

Notes:

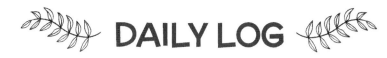

DAILY LOG

Date: ___/___/_____   M T W Th F Sa Su

Breakfast

Meal	Calories	Fat (g)	Carbs (g)	Sugar (g)	Fiber (g)	Net Carb (carbs-fiber)	Protein (g)	Sodium (mg)
Totals:								

Blood Glucose Levels			Blood Pressure Levels		Insulin/Medications		
Before:		Time:	(systolic):	Heart Rate (per min)	Type/Units	Pre	Post
After:		Time:	(diastolic):				

Snack #1

Totals:								

Blood Glucose Levels			Blood Pressure Levels		Insulin/Medications		
Before:		Time:	(systolic):	Heart Rate (per min)	Type/Units	Pre	Post
After:		Time:	(diastolic):				

Lunch

Totals:								

Blood Glucose Levels			Blood Pressure Levels		Insulin/Medications		
Before:		Time:	(systolic):	Heart Rate (per min)	Type/Units	Pre	Post
After:		Time:	(diastolic):				

Snack #2

Totals:								

Blood Glucose Levels			Blood Pressure Levels		Insulin/Medications		
Before:		Time:	(systolic):	Heart Rate (per min)	Type/Units	Pre	Post
After:		Time:	(diastolic):				

Dinner

Totals:								

Blood Glucose Levels			Blood Pressure Levels		Insulin/Medications		
Before:		Time:	(systolic):	Heart Rate (per min)	Type/Units	Pre	Post
After:		Time:	(diastolic):				

Fasting Blood Sugar:

_____

Water Intake:

total ounces _____

Fitness Log:

Activity	Min

Sleep Log:

Total Hours _____

Notes:

_____
_____
_____
_____
_____
_____
_____
_____
_____
_____
_____

DAILY LOG

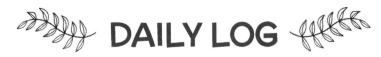

Date: ___/___/_____   **M T W Th F Sa Su**

Breakfast

	Meal	Calories	Fat (g)	Carbs (g)	Sugar (g)	Fiber (g)	Net Carb (carbs-fiber)	Protein (g)	Sodium (mg)
	Totals:								

Blood Glucose Levels				Blood Pressure Levels			Insulin/Medications		
Before:		Time:		(systolic):		Heart Rate (per min)	Type/Units	Pre	Post
After:		Time:		(diastolic):					

Snack #1

	Meal	Calories	Fat (g)	Carbs (g)	Sugar (g)	Fiber (g)	Net Carb (carbs-fiber)	Protein (g)	Sodium (mg)
	Totals:								

Blood Glucose Levels				Blood Pressure Levels			Insulin/Medications		
Before:		Time:		(systolic):		Heart Rate (per min)	Type/Units	Pre	Post
After:		Time:		(diastolic):					

Lunch

	Meal	Calories	Fat (g)	Carbs (g)	Sugar (g)	Fiber (g)	Net Carb (carbs-fiber)	Protein (g)	Sodium (mg)
	Totals:								

Blood Glucose Levels				Blood Pressure Levels			Insulin/Medications		
Before:		Time:		(systolic):		Heart Rate (per min)	Type/Units	Pre	Post
After:		Time:		(diastolic):					

Snack #2

	Meal	Calories	Fat (g)	Carbs (g)	Sugar (g)	Fiber (g)	Net Carb (carbs-fiber)	Protein (g)	Sodium (mg)
	Totals:								

Blood Glucose Levels				Blood Pressure Levels			Insulin/Medications		
Before:		Time:		(systolic):		Heart Rate (per min)	Type/Units	Pre	Post
After:		Time:		(diastolic):					

Dinner

	Meal	Calories	Fat (g)	Carbs (g)	Sugar (g)	Fiber (g)	Net Carb (carbs-fiber)	Protein (g)	Sodium (mg)
	Totals:								

Blood Glucose Levels				Blood Pressure Levels			Insulin/Medications		
Before:		Time:		(systolic):		Heart Rate (per min)	Type/Units	Pre	Post
After:		Time:		(diastolic):					

Fasting Blood Sugar:

_____

Water Intake:

total ounces _____

Fitness Log:

Activity   Min

Sleep Log:

Total Hours _____

Notes:

DAILY LOG

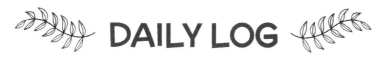

Date: ___/___/_____   **M T W Th F Sa Su**

Breakfast

Meal	Calories	Fat (g)	Carbs (g)	Sugar (g)	Fiber (g)	Net Carb (carbs-fiber)	Protein (g)	Sodium (mg)
Totals:								

Blood Glucose Levels			Blood Pressure Levels		Insulin/Medications		
Before:		Time:		Heart Rate (per min)	Type/Units	Pre	Post
After:		Time:	(systolic):				
			(diastolic):				

Snack #1

Totals:								

Blood Glucose Levels			Blood Pressure Levels		Insulin/Medications		
Before:		Time:		Heart Rate (per min)	Type/Units	Pre	Post
After:		Time:	(systolic):				
			(diastolic):				

Lunch

Totals:								

Blood Glucose Levels			Blood Pressure Levels		Insulin/Medications		
Before:		Time:		Heart Rate (per min)	Type/Units	Pre	Post
After:		Time:	(systolic):				
			(diastolic):				

Snack #2

Totals:								

Blood Glucose Levels			Blood Pressure Levels		Insulin/Medications		
Before:		Time:		Heart Rate (per min)	Type/Units	Pre	Post
After:		Time:	(systolic):				
			(diastolic):				

Dinner

Totals:								

Blood Glucose Levels			Blood Pressure Levels		Insulin/Medications		
Before:		Time:		Heart Rate (per min)	Type/Units	Pre	Post
After:		Time:	(systolic):				
			(diastolic):				

Fasting Blood Sugar:

_____

Water Intake:

total ounces _____

Fitness Log:

Activity	Min

Sleep Log:

Total Hours _____

Notes:

DAILY LOG

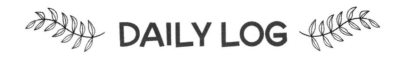

Date: ___/___/_____   **M T W Th F Sa Su**

Breakfast

Meal	Calories	Fat (g)	Carbs (g)	Sugar (g)	Fiber (g)	Net Carb (carbs-fiber)	Protein (g)	Sodium (mg)
Totals:								

Blood Glucose Levels				Blood Pressure Levels		Insulin/Medications		
					Heart Rate (per min)	Type/Units	Pre	Post
Before:		Time:		(systolic):				
After:		Time:		(diastolic):				

Snack #1

Totals:								

Blood Glucose Levels				Blood Pressure Levels		Insulin/Medications		
					Heart Rate (per min)	Type/Units	Pre	Post
Before:		Time:		(systolic):				
After:		Time:		(diastolic):				

Lunch

Totals:								

Blood Glucose Levels				Blood Pressure Levels		Insulin/Medications		
					Heart Rate (per min)	Type/Units	Pre	Post
Before:		Time:		(systolic):				
After:		Time:		(diastolic):				

Snack #2

Totals:								

Blood Glucose Levels				Blood Pressure Levels		Insulin/Medications		
					Heart Rate (per min)	Type/Units	Pre	Post
Before:		Time:		(systolic):				
After:		Time:		(diastolic):				

Dinner

Totals:								

Blood Glucose Levels				Blood Pressure Levels		Insulin/Medications		
					Heart Rate (per min)	Type/Units	Pre	Post
Before:		Time:		(systolic):				
After:		Time:		(diastolic):				

Fasting Blood Sugar:
_____

Water Intake:
total ounces _____

Fitness Log:

Activity	Min

Sleep Log:
Total Hours _____

Notes:
_____
_____
_____
_____
_____
_____
_____
_____
_____
_____

DAILY LOG

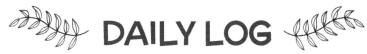

Date: ___/___/_____   **M T W Th F Sa Su**

Breakfast

Meal	Calories	Fat (g)	Carbs (g)	Sugar (g)	Fiber (g)	Net Carb (carbs-fiber)	Protein (g)	Sodium (mg)
Totals:								

Blood Glucose Levels			Blood Pressure Levels		Insulin/Medications		
Before:		Time:	(systolic):	Heart Rate (per min)	Type/Units	Pre	Post
After:		Time:	(diastolic):				

Snack #1

Totals:								

Blood Glucose Levels			Blood Pressure Levels		Insulin/Medications		
Before:		Time:	(systolic):	Heart Rate (per min)	Type/Units	Pre	Post
After:		Time:	(diastolic):				

Lunch

Totals:								

Blood Glucose Levels			Blood Pressure Levels		Insulin/Medications		
Before:		Time:	(systolic):	Heart Rate (per min)	Type/Units	Pre	Post
After:		Time:	(diastolic):				

Snack #2

Totals:								

Blood Glucose Levels			Blood Pressure Levels		Insulin/Medications		
Before:		Time:	(systolic):	Heart Rate (per min)	Type/Units	Pre	Post
After:		Time:	(diastolic):				

Dinner

Totals:								

Blood Glucose Levels			Blood Pressure Levels		Insulin/Medications		
Before:		Time:	(systolic):	Heart Rate (per min)	Type/Units	Pre	Post
After:		Time:	(diastolic):				

Fasting Blood Sugar:
_____

Water Intake:
total ounces _____

Fitness Log:
Activity	Min

Sleep Log:
Total Hours _____

Notes:
_____
_____
_____
_____
_____
_____
_____
_____
_____
_____

DAILY LOG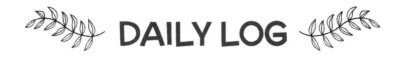

Date: ___/___/_____   M T W Th F Sa Su

Breakfast

Meal	Calories	Fat (g)	Carbs (g)	Sugar (g)	Fiber (g)	Net Carb (carbs-fiber)	Protein (g)	Sodium (mg)
Totals:								

Blood Glucose Levels				Blood Pressure Levels		Heart Rate (per min)	Insulin/Medications		
Before:		Time:		(systolic):			Type/Units	Pre	Post
After:		Time:		(diastolic):					

Snack #1

Totals:								

Blood Glucose Levels				Blood Pressure Levels		Heart Rate (per min)	Insulin/Medications		
Before:		Time:		(systolic):			Type/Units	Pre	Post
After:		Time:		(diastolic):					

Lunch

Totals:								

Blood Glucose Levels				Blood Pressure Levels		Heart Rate (per min)	Insulin/Medications		
Before:		Time:		(systolic):			Type/Units	Pre	Post
After:		Time:		(diastolic):					

Snack #2

Totals:								

Blood Glucose Levels				Blood Pressure Levels		Heart Rate (per min)	Insulin/Medications		
Before:		Time:		(systolic):			Type/Units	Pre	Post
After:		Time:		(diastolic):					

Dinner

Totals:								

Blood Glucose Levels				Blood Pressure Levels		Heart Rate (per min)	Insulin/Medications		
Before:		Time:		(systolic):			Type/Units	Pre	Post
After:		Time:		(diastolic):					

Fasting Blood Sugar:

_____

Water Intake:

total ounces _____

Fitness Log:

Activity	Min

Sleep Log:

Total Hours _____

Notes:

_____
_____
_____
_____
_____
_____
_____
_____
_____
_____
_____

DAILY LOG

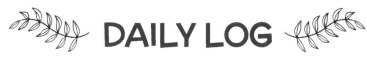

Date: ____/____/_____

M T W Th F Sa Su

Breakfast

Meal	Calories	Fat (g)	Carbs (g)	Sugar (g)	Fiber (g)	Net Carb (carbs-fiber)	Protein (g)	Sodium (mg)
Totals:								

Blood Glucose Levels				Blood Pressure Levels			Insulin/Medications		
Before:		Time:		(systolic):		Heart Rate (per min)	Type/Units	Pre	Post
After:		Time:		(diastolic):					

Snack #1

Totals:								

Blood Glucose Levels				Blood Pressure Levels			Insulin/Medications		
Before:		Time:		(systolic):		Heart Rate (per min)	Type/Units	Pre	Post
After:		Time:		(diastolic):					

Lunch

Totals:								

Blood Glucose Levels				Blood Pressure Levels			Insulin/Medications		
Before:		Time:		(systolic):		Heart Rate (per min)	Type/Units	Pre	Post
After:		Time:		(diastolic):					

Snack #2

Totals:								

Blood Glucose Levels				Blood Pressure Levels			Insulin/Medications		
Before:		Time:		(systolic):		Heart Rate (per min)	Type/Units	Pre	Post
After:		Time:		(diastolic):					

Dinner

Totals:								

Blood Glucose Levels				Blood Pressure Levels			Insulin/Medications		
Before:		Time:		(systolic):		Heart Rate (per min)	Type/Units	Pre	Post
After:		Time:		(diastolic):					

Fasting Blood Sugar:

_____

Water Intake:

total ounces _____

Fitness Log:

Activity	Min

Sleep Log:

Total Hours _____

Notes:

_____
_____
_____
_____
_____
_____
_____
_____
_____
_____
_____

DAILY LOG

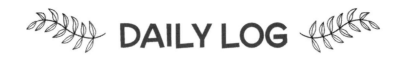

Date: ____/____/_____   **M T W Th F Sa Su**

Breakfast

Meal	Calories	Fat (g)	Carbs (g)	Sugar (g)	Fiber (g)	Net Carb (carbs-fiber)	Protein (g)	Sodium (mg)
Totals:								

Blood Glucose Levels				Blood Pressure Levels			Insulin/Medications		
						Heart Rate (per min)	Type/Units	Pre	Post
Before:		Time:		(systolic):					
After:		Time:		(diastolic):					

Snack #1

Totals:								

Blood Glucose Levels				Blood Pressure Levels			Insulin/Medications		
						Heart Rate (per min)	Type/Units	Pre	Post
Before:		Time:		(systolic):					
After:		Time:		(diastolic):					

Lunch

Totals:								

Blood Glucose Levels				Blood Pressure Levels			Insulin/Medications		
						Heart Rate (per min)	Type/Units	Pre	Post
Before:		Time:		(systolic):					
After:		Time:		(diastolic):					

Snack #2

Totals:								

Blood Glucose Levels				Blood Pressure Levels			Insulin/Medications		
						Heart Rate (per min)	Type/Units	Pre	Post
Before:		Time:		(systolic):					
After:		Time:		(diastolic):					

Dinner

Totals:								

Blood Glucose Levels				Blood Pressure Levels			Insulin/Medications		
						Heart Rate (per min)	Type/Units	Pre	Post
Before:		Time:		(systolic):					
After:		Time:		(diastolic):					

Fasting Blood Sugar:

_____

Water Intake:

total ounces _____

Fitness Log:

Activity	Min

Sleep Log:

Total Hours _____

Notes:

DAILY LOG

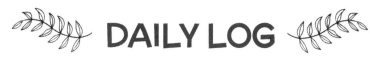

Date: ___/___/_____   **M   T   W   Th   F   Sa   Su**

Breakfast

Meal	Calories	Fat (g)	Carbs (g)	Sugar (g)	Fiber (g)	Net Carb (carbs-fiber)	Protein (g)	Sodium (mg)
Totals:								

Blood Glucose Levels			Blood Pressure Levels			Insulin/Medications		
Before:		Time:	(systolic):		Heart Rate (per min)	Type/Units	Pre	Post
After:		Time:	(diastolic):					

Snack #1

Totals:								

Blood Glucose Levels			Blood Pressure Levels			Insulin/Medications		
Before:		Time:	(systolic):		Heart Rate (per min)	Type/Units	Pre	Post
After:		Time:	(diastolic):					

Lunch

Totals:								

Blood Glucose Levels			Blood Pressure Levels			Insulin/Medications		
Before:		Time:	(systolic):		Heart Rate (per min)	Type/Units	Pre	Post
After:		Time:	(diastolic):					

Snack #2

Totals:								

Blood Glucose Levels			Blood Pressure Levels			Insulin/Medications		
Before:		Time:	(systolic):		Heart Rate (per min)	Type/Units	Pre	Post
After:		Time:	(diastolic):					

Dinner

Totals:								

Blood Glucose Levels			Blood Pressure Levels			Insulin/Medications		
Before:		Time:	(systolic):		Heart Rate (per min)	Type/Units	Pre	Post
After:		Time:	(diastolic):					

Fasting Blood Sugar:
_____

Water Intake:
total ounces _____

Fitness Log:
Activity	Min

Sleep Log:
Total Hours _____

Notes:
_____
_____
_____
_____
_____
_____
_____
_____
_____
_____

DAILY LOG

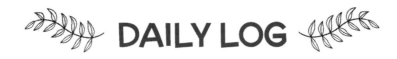

Date: ___/___/_____   **M T W Th F Sa Su**

Breakfast

	Meal	Calories	Fat (g)	Carbs (g)	Sugar (g)	Fiber (g)	Net Carb (carbs-fiber)	Protein (g)	Sodium (mg)
	Totals:								

Blood Glucose Levels				Blood Pressure Levels			Insulin/Medications		
Before:		Time:		(systolic):		Heart Rate (per min)	Type/Units	Pre	Post
After:		Time:		(diastolic):					

Snack #1

	Totals:								

Blood Glucose Levels				Blood Pressure Levels			Insulin/Medications		
Before:		Time:		(systolic):		Heart Rate (per min)	Type/Units	Pre	Post
After:		Time:		(diastolic):					

Lunch

	Totals:								

Blood Glucose Levels				Blood Pressure Levels			Insulin/Medications		
Before:		Time:		(systolic):		Heart Rate (per min)	Type/Units	Pre	Post
After:		Time:		(diastolic):					

Snack #2

	Totals:								

Blood Glucose Levels				Blood Pressure Levels			Insulin/Medications		
Before:		Time:		(systolic):		Heart Rate (per min)	Type/Units	Pre	Post
After:		Time:		(diastolic):					

Dinner

	Totals:								

Blood Glucose Levels				Blood Pressure Levels			Insulin/Medications		
Before:		Time:		(systolic):		Heart Rate (per min)	Type/Units	Pre	Post
After:		Time:		(diastolic):					

Fasting Blood Sugar:

_____

Water Intake:

total ounces _____

Fitness Log:

Activity	Min

Sleep Log:

Total Hours _____

Notes:

_____
_____
_____
_____
_____
_____
_____
_____
_____
_____

DAILY LOG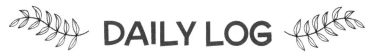

Date: ___/___/_____   M T W Th F Sa Su

Breakfast

	Meal	Calories	Fat (g)	Carbs (g)	Sugar (g)	Fiber (g)	Net Carb (carbs-fiber)	Protein (g)	Sodium (mg)
	Totals:								

Blood Glucose Levels			Blood Pressure Levels		Insulin/Medications		
Before:		Time:	(systolic):	Heart Rate (per min)	Type/Units	Pre	Post
After:		Time:	(diastolic):				

Fasting Blood Sugar:

_____

Snack #1

	Totals:								

Blood Glucose Levels			Blood Pressure Levels		Insulin/Medications		
Before:		Time:	(systolic):	Heart Rate (per min)	Type/Units	Pre	Post
After:		Time:	(diastolic):				

Water Intake:

total ounces _____

Lunch

	Totals:								

Blood Glucose Levels			Blood Pressure Levels		Insulin/Medications		
Before:		Time:	(systolic):	Heart Rate (per min)	Type/Units	Pre	Post
After:		Time:	(diastolic):				

Fitness Log:

Activity   Min

Sleep Log:

Total Hours _____

Snack #2

	Totals:								

Blood Glucose Levels			Blood Pressure Levels		Insulin/Medications		
Before:		Time:	(systolic):	Heart Rate (per min)	Type/Units	Pre	Post
After:		Time:	(diastolic):				

Notes:

Dinner

	Totals:								

Blood Glucose Levels			Blood Pressure Levels		Insulin/Medications		
Before:		Time:	(systolic):	Heart Rate (per min)	Type/Units	Pre	Post
After:		Time:	(diastolic):				

DAILY LOG

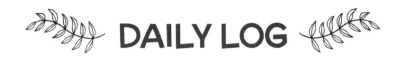

Date: ___/___/_____   **M T W Th F Sa Su**

Breakfast

	Meal	Calories	Fat (g)	Carbs (g)	Sugar (g)	Fiber (g)	Net Carb (carbs-fiber)	Protein (g)	Sodium (mg)
	Totals:								

Blood Glucose Levels				Blood Pressure Levels			Insulin/Medications		
Before:		Time:		(systolic):		Heart Rate (per min)	Type/Units	Pre	Post
After:		Time:		(diastolic):					

Snack #1

	Totals:								

Blood Glucose Levels				Blood Pressure Levels			Insulin/Medications		
Before:		Time:		(systolic):		Heart Rate (per min)	Type/Units	Pre	Post
After:		Time:		(diastolic):					

Lunch

	Totals:								

Blood Glucose Levels				Blood Pressure Levels			Insulin/Medications		
Before:		Time:		(systolic):		Heart Rate (per min)	Type/Units	Pre	Post
After:		Time:		(diastolic):					

Snack #2

	Totals:								

Blood Glucose Levels				Blood Pressure Levels			Insulin/Medications		
Before:		Time:		(systolic):		Heart Rate (per min)	Type/Units	Pre	Post
After:		Time:		(diastolic):					

Dinner

	Totals:								

Blood Glucose Levels				Blood Pressure Levels			Insulin/Medications		
Before:		Time:		(systolic):		Heart Rate (per min)	Type/Units	Pre	Post
After:		Time:		(diastolic):					

Fasting Blood Sugar:

_____

Water Intake:

total ounces _____

Fitness Log:

Activity	Min

Sleep Log:

Total Hours _____

Notes:

_____
_____
_____
_____
_____
_____
_____
_____
_____
_____

DAILY LOG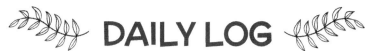

Date: ___/___/_____   **M T W Th F Sa Su**

Breakfast

	Meal	Calories	Fat (g)	Carbs (g)	Sugar (g)	Fiber (g)	Net Carb (carbs-fiber)	Protein (g)	Sodium (mg)
Totals:									

Blood Glucose Levels			Blood Pressure Levels		Insulin/Medications		
Before:		Time:	(systolic):	Heart Rate (per min)	Type/Units	Pre	Post
After:		Time:	(diastolic):				

Snack #1

Totals:									

Blood Glucose Levels			Blood Pressure Levels		Insulin/Medications		
Before:		Time:	(systolic):	Heart Rate (per min)	Type/Units	Pre	Post
After:		Time:	(diastolic):				

Lunch

Totals:									

Blood Glucose Levels			Blood Pressure Levels		Insulin/Medications		
Before:		Time:	(systolic):	Heart Rate (per min)	Type/Units	Pre	Post
After:		Time:	(diastolic):				

Snack #2

Totals:									

Blood Glucose Levels			Blood Pressure Levels		Insulin/Medications		
Before:		Time:	(systolic):	Heart Rate (per min)	Type/Units	Pre	Post
After:		Time:	(diastolic):				

Dinner

Totals:									

Blood Glucose Levels			Blood Pressure Levels		Insulin/Medications		
Before:		Time:	(systolic):	Heart Rate (per min)	Type/Units	Pre	Post
After:		Time:	(diastolic):				

Fasting Blood Sugar:

_____

Water Intake:

total ounces _____

Fitness Log:

Activity	Min

Sleep Log:

Total Hours _____

Notes:

_____
_____
_____
_____
_____
_____
_____
_____
_____

DAILY LOG

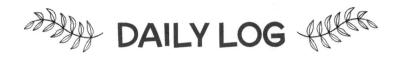

Date: ___/___/_____   **M T W Th F Sa Su**

Breakfast

	Meal	Calories	Fat (g)	Carbs (g)	Sugar (g)	Fiber (g)	Net Carb (carbs-fiber)	Protein (g)	Sodium (mg)
	Totals:								

Blood Glucose Levels			Blood Pressure Levels		Insulin/Medications		
Before:		Time:	(systolic):	Heart Rate (per min)	Type/Units	Pre	Post
After:		Time:	(diastolic):				

Snack #1

	Totals:								

Blood Glucose Levels			Blood Pressure Levels		Insulin/Medications		
Before:		Time:	(systolic):	Heart Rate (per min)	Type/Units	Pre	Post
After:		Time:	(diastolic):				

Lunch

	Totals:								

Blood Glucose Levels			Blood Pressure Levels		Insulin/Medications		
Before:		Time:	(systolic):	Heart Rate (per min)	Type/Units	Pre	Post
After:		Time:	(diastolic):				

Snack #2

	Totals:								

Blood Glucose Levels			Blood Pressure Levels		Insulin/Medications		
Before:		Time:	(systolic):	Heart Rate (per min)	Type/Units	Pre	Post
After:		Time:	(diastolic):				

Dinner

	Totals:								

Blood Glucose Levels			Blood Pressure Levels		Insulin/Medications		
Before:		Time:	(systolic):	Heart Rate (per min)	Type/Units	Pre	Post
After:		Time:	(diastolic):				

Fasting Blood Sugar:

_____

Water Intake:

total ounces _____

Fitness Log:

Activity	Min

Sleep Log:

Total Hours _____

Notes:

_____
_____
_____
_____
_____
_____
_____
_____
_____

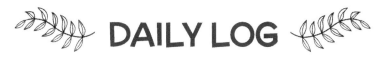

DAILY LOG

Date: ___/___/_____   M T W Th F Sa Su

Breakfast

	Meal	Calories	Fat (g)	Carbs (g)	Sugar (g)	Fiber (g)	Net Carb (carbs-fiber)	Protein (g)	Sodium (mg)
	Totals:								

Blood Glucose Levels			Blood Pressure Levels		Insulin/Medications		
Before:		Time:	(systolic):	Heart Rate (per min)	Type/Units	Pre	Post
After:		Time:	(diastolic):				

Snack #1

	Totals:								

Blood Glucose Levels			Blood Pressure Levels		Insulin/Medications		
Before:		Time:	(systolic):	Heart Rate (per min)	Type/Units	Pre	Post
After:		Time:	(diastolic):				

Lunch

	Totals:								

Blood Glucose Levels			Blood Pressure Levels		Insulin/Medications		
Before:		Time:	(systolic):	Heart Rate (per min)	Type/Units	Pre	Post
After:		Time:	(diastolic):				

Snack #2

	Totals:								

Blood Glucose Levels			Blood Pressure Levels		Insulin/Medications		
Before:		Time:	(systolic):	Heart Rate (per min)	Type/Units	Pre	Post
After:		Time:	(diastolic):				

Dinner

	Totals:								

Blood Glucose Levels			Blood Pressure Levels		Insulin/Medications		
Before:		Time:	(systolic):	Heart Rate (per min)	Type/Units	Pre	Post
After:		Time:	(diastolic):				

Fasting Blood Sugar:

_____

Water Intake:

total ounces _____

Fitness Log:

Activity	Min

Sleep Log:

Total Hours _____

Notes:

DAILY LOG

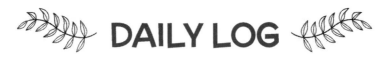

Date: ___/___/_____   **M T W Th F Sa Su**

Breakfast

	Meal	Calories	Fat (g)	Carbs (g)	Sugar (g)	Fiber (g)	Net Carb (carbs-fiber)	Protein (g)	Sodium (mg)
	Totals:								

Blood Glucose Levels		Blood Pressure Levels		Insulin/Medications		
			Heart Rate (per min)	Type/Units	Pre	Post
Before:	Time:	(systolic):				
After:	Time:	(diastolic):				

Snack #1

	Totals:								

Blood Glucose Levels		Blood Pressure Levels		Insulin/Medications		
			Heart Rate (per min)	Type/Units	Pre	Post
Before:	Time:	(systolic):				
After:	Time:	(diastolic):				

Lunch

	Totals:								

Blood Glucose Levels		Blood Pressure Levels		Insulin/Medications		
			Heart Rate (per min)	Type/Units	Pre	Post
Before:	Time:	(systolic):				
After:	Time:	(diastolic):				

Snack #2

	Totals:								

Blood Glucose Levels		Blood Pressure Levels		Insulin/Medications		
			Heart Rate (per min)	Type/Units	Pre	Post
Before:	Time:	(systolic):				
After:	Time:	(diastolic):				

Dinner

	Totals:								

Blood Glucose Levels		Blood Pressure Levels		Insulin/Medications		
			Heart Rate (per min)	Type/Units	Pre	Post
Before:	Time:	(systolic):				
After:	Time:	(diastolic):				

Fasting Blood Sugar:

_____

Water Intake:

total ounces _____

Fitness Log:

Activity	Min

Sleep Log:

Total Hours _____

Notes:

DAILY LOG

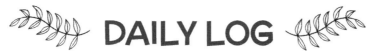

Date: ___/___/_____   **M T W Th F Sa Su**

Breakfast

Meal	Calories	Fat (g)	Carbs (g)	Sugar (g)	Fiber (g)	Net Carb (carbs-fiber)	Protein (g)	Sodium (mg)
Totals:								

Blood Glucose Levels			Blood Pressure Levels			Insulin/Medications		
Before:		Time:	(systolic):		Heart Rate (per min)	Type/Units	Pre	Post
After:		Time:	(diastolic):					

Snack #1

Totals:								

Blood Glucose Levels			Blood Pressure Levels			Insulin/Medications		
Before:		Time:	(systolic):		Heart Rate (per min)	Type/Units	Pre	Post
After:		Time:	(diastolic):					

Lunch

Totals:								

Blood Glucose Levels			Blood Pressure Levels			Insulin/Medications		
Before:		Time:	(systolic):		Heart Rate (per min)	Type/Units	Pre	Post
After:		Time:	(diastolic):					

Snack #2

Totals:								

Blood Glucose Levels			Blood Pressure Levels			Insulin/Medications		
Before:		Time:	(systolic):		Heart Rate (per min)	Type/Units	Pre	Post
After:		Time:	(diastolic):					

Dinner

Totals:								

Blood Glucose Levels			Blood Pressure Levels			Insulin/Medications		
Before:		Time:	(systolic):		Heart Rate (per min)	Type/Units	Pre	Post
After:		Time:	(diastolic):					

Fasting Blood Sugar:

_____

Water Intake:

total ounces _____

Fitness Log:

Activity	Min

Sleep Log:

Total Hours _____

Notes:

DAILY LOG
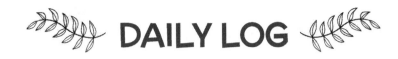

Date: ___/___/_____   M T W Th F Sa Su

Breakfast

Meal	Calories	Fat (g)	Carbs (g)	Sugar (g)	Fiber (g)	Net Carb (carbs-fiber)	Protein (g)	Sodium (mg)
Totals:								

Blood Glucose Levels			Blood Pressure Levels		Insulin/Medications		
				Heart Rate (per min)	Type/Units	Pre	Post
Before:		Time:	(systolic):				
After:		Time:	(diastolic):				

Snack #1

Totals:								

Blood Glucose Levels			Blood Pressure Levels		Insulin/Medications		
				Heart Rate (per min)	Type/Units	Pre	Post
Before:		Time:	(systolic):				
After:		Time:	(diastolic):				

Lunch

Totals:								

Blood Glucose Levels			Blood Pressure Levels		Insulin/Medications		
				Heart Rate (per min)	Type/Units	Pre	Post
Before:		Time:	(systolic):				
After:		Time:	(diastolic):				

Snack #2

Totals:								

Blood Glucose Levels			Blood Pressure Levels		Insulin/Medications		
				Heart Rate (per min)	Type/Units	Pre	Post
Before:		Time:	(systolic):				
After:		Time:	(diastolic):				

Dinner

Totals:								

Blood Glucose Levels			Blood Pressure Levels		Insulin/Medications		
				Heart Rate (per min)	Type/Units	Pre	Post
Before:		Time:	(systolic):				
After:		Time:	(diastolic):				

Fasting Blood Sugar:
_____

Water Intake:
total ounces _____

Fitness Log:

Activity	Min

Sleep Log:
Total Hours _____

Notes:
_____
_____
_____
_____
_____
_____
_____
_____
_____
_____
_____
_____

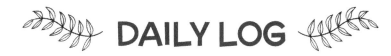

DAILY LOG

Date: ___/___/_____

M T W Th F Sa Su

Breakfast

Meal	Calories	Fat (g)	Carbs (g)	Sugar (g)	Fiber (g)	Net Carb (carbs-fiber)	Protein (g)	Sodium (mg)
Totals:								

Blood Glucose Levels				Blood Pressure Levels			Insulin/Medications		
Before:		Time:		(systolic):		Heart Rate (per min)	Type/Units	Pre	Post
After:		Time:		(diastolic):					

Snack #1

Totals:								

Blood Glucose Levels				Blood Pressure Levels			Insulin/Medications		
Before:		Time:		(systolic):		Heart Rate (per min)	Type/Units	Pre	Post
After:		Time:		(diastolic):					

Lunch

Totals:								

Blood Glucose Levels				Blood Pressure Levels			Insulin/Medications		
Before:		Time:		(systolic):		Heart Rate (per min)	Type/Units	Pre	Post
After:		Time:		(diastolic):					

Snack #2

Totals:								

Blood Glucose Levels				Blood Pressure Levels			Insulin/Medications		
Before:		Time:		(systolic):		Heart Rate (per min)	Type/Units	Pre	Post
After:		Time:		(diastolic):					

Dinner

Totals:								

Blood Glucose Levels				Blood Pressure Levels			Insulin/Medications		
Before:		Time:		(systolic):		Heart Rate (per min)	Type/Units	Pre	Post
After:		Time:		(diastolic):					

Fasting Blood Sugar:

_____

Water Intake:

total ounces _____

Fitness Log:

Activity	Min

Sleep Log:

Total Hours _____

Notes:

_____
_____
_____
_____
_____
_____
_____
_____
_____
_____

DAILY LOG

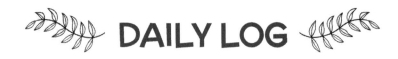

Date: ___/___/_____

M T W Th F Sa Su

Breakfast

	Meal	Calories	Fat (g)	Carbs (g)	Sugar (g)	Fiber (g)	Net Carb (carbs-fiber)	Protein (g)	Sodium (mg)
	Totals:								

Blood Glucose Levels				Blood Pressure Levels			Insulin/Medications		
Before:		Time:		(systolic):		Heart Rate (per min)	Type/Units	Pre	Post
After:		Time:		(diastolic):					

Snack #1

	Totals:								

Blood Glucose Levels				Blood Pressure Levels			Insulin/Medications		
Before:		Time:		(systolic):		Heart Rate (per min)	Type/Units	Pre	Post
After:		Time:		(diastolic):					

Lunch

	Totals:								

Blood Glucose Levels				Blood Pressure Levels			Insulin/Medications		
Before:		Time:		(systolic):		Heart Rate (per min)	Type/Units	Pre	Post
After:		Time:		(diastolic):					

Snack #2

	Totals:								

Blood Glucose Levels				Blood Pressure Levels			Insulin/Medications		
Before:		Time:		(systolic):		Heart Rate (per min)	Type/Units	Pre	Post
After:		Time:		(diastolic):					

Dinner

	Totals:								

Blood Glucose Levels				Blood Pressure Levels			Insulin/Medications		
Before:		Time:		(systolic):		Heart Rate (per min)	Type/Units	Pre	Post
After:		Time:		(diastolic):					

Fasting Blood Sugar:

_____

Water Intake:

total ounces _____

Fitness Log:

Activity	Min

Sleep Log:

Total Hours _____

Notes:

DAILY LOG

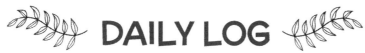

Date: ___/___/_____   **M T W Th F Sa Su**

Breakfast

	Meal	Calories	Fat (g)	Carbs (g)	Sugar (g)	Fiber (g)	Net Carb (carbs-fiber)	Protein (g)	Sodium (mg)
	Totals:								

Blood Glucose Levels				Blood Pressure Levels			Insulin/Medications		
Before:		Time:		(systolic):		Heart Rate (per min)	Type/Units	Pre	Post
After:		Time:		(diastolic):					

Snack #1

	Totals:								

Blood Glucose Levels				Blood Pressure Levels			Insulin/Medications		
Before:		Time:		(systolic):		Heart Rate (per min)	Type/Units	Pre	Post
After:		Time:		(diastolic):					

Lunch

	Totals:								

Blood Glucose Levels				Blood Pressure Levels			Insulin/Medications		
Before:		Time:		(systolic):		Heart Rate (per min)	Type/Units	Pre	Post
After:		Time:		(diastolic):					

Snack #2

	Totals:								

Blood Glucose Levels				Blood Pressure Levels			Insulin/Medications		
Before:		Time:		(systolic):		Heart Rate (per min)	Type/Units	Pre	Post
After:		Time:		(diastolic):					

Dinner

	Totals:								

Blood Glucose Levels				Blood Pressure Levels			Insulin/Medications		
Before:		Time:		(systolic):		Heart Rate (per min)	Type/Units	Pre	Post
After:		Time:		(diastolic):					

Fasting Blood Sugar:

_____

Water Intake:

total ounces _____

Fitness Log:

Activity	Min

Sleep Log:

Total Hours _____

Notes:

DAILY LOG

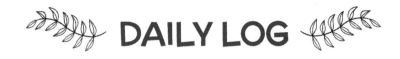

Date: ___/___/_____   **M T W Th F Sa Su**

Breakfast

Meal	Calories	Fat (g)	Carbs (g)	Sugar (g)	Fiber (g)	Net Carb (carbs-fiber)	Protein (g)	Sodium (mg)
Totals:								

Blood Glucose Levels			Blood Pressure Levels		Insulin/Medications		
Before:		Time:	(systolic):	Heart Rate (per min)	Type/Units	Pre	Post
After:		Time:	(diastolic):				

Snack #1

Totals:								

Blood Glucose Levels			Blood Pressure Levels		Insulin/Medications		
Before:		Time:	(systolic):	Heart Rate (per min)	Type/Units	Pre	Post
After:		Time:	(diastolic):				

Lunch

Totals:								

Blood Glucose Levels			Blood Pressure Levels		Insulin/Medications		
Before:		Time:	(systolic):	Heart Rate (per min)	Type/Units	Pre	Post
After:		Time:	(diastolic):				

Snack #2

Totals:								

Blood Glucose Levels			Blood Pressure Levels		Insulin/Medications		
Before:		Time:	(systolic):	Heart Rate (per min)	Type/Units	Pre	Post
After:		Time:	(diastolic):				

Dinner

Totals:								

Blood Glucose Levels			Blood Pressure Levels		Insulin/Medications		
Before:		Time:	(systolic):	Heart Rate (per min)	Type/Units	Pre	Post
After:		Time:	(diastolic):				

Fasting Blood Sugar:

_____

Water Intake:

total ounces _____

Fitness Log:

Activity	Min

Sleep Log:

Total Hours _____

Notes:

DAILY LOG

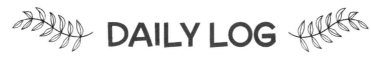

Date: ___/___/_____   M T W Th F Sa Su

Breakfast

Meal	Calories	Fat (g)	Carbs (g)	Sugar (g)	Fiber (g)	Net Carb (carbs-fiber)	Protein (g)	Sodium (mg)
Totals:								

Blood Glucose Levels			Blood Pressure Levels			Insulin/Medications		
Before:		Time:	(systolic):		Heart Rate (per min)	Type/Units	Pre	Post
After:		Time:	(diastolic):					

Snack #1

Totals:								

Blood Glucose Levels			Blood Pressure Levels			Insulin/Medications		
Before:		Time:	(systolic):		Heart Rate (per min)	Type/Units	Pre	Post
After:		Time:	(diastolic):					

Lunch

Totals:								

Blood Glucose Levels			Blood Pressure Levels			Insulin/Medications		
Before:		Time:	(systolic):		Heart Rate (per min)	Type/Units	Pre	Post
After:		Time:	(diastolic):					

Snack #2

Totals:								

Blood Glucose Levels			Blood Pressure Levels			Insulin/Medications		
Before:		Time:	(systolic):		Heart Rate (per min)	Type/Units	Pre	Post
After:		Time:	(diastolic):					

Dinner

Totals:								

Blood Glucose Levels			Blood Pressure Levels			Insulin/Medications		
Before:		Time:	(systolic):		Heart Rate (per min)	Type/Units	Pre	Post
After:		Time:	(diastolic):					

Fasting Blood Sugar:
_____

Water Intake:
total ounces _____

Fitness Log:
Activity	Min

Sleep Log:
Total Hours _____

Notes:
_____
_____
_____
_____
_____
_____
_____
_____
_____

DAILY LOG

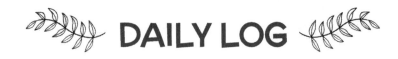

Date: ___/___/_____   M T W Th F Sa Su

Breakfast

	Meal	Calories	Fat (g)	Carbs (g)	Sugar (g)	Fiber (g)	Net Carb (carbs-fiber)	Protein (g)	Sodium (mg)
	Totals:								

Blood Glucose Levels				Blood Pressure Levels			Insulin/Medications		
Before:		Time:		(systolic):		Heart Rate (per min)	Type/Units	Pre	Post
After:		Time:		(diastolic):					

Snack #1

	Totals:								

Blood Glucose Levels				Blood Pressure Levels			Insulin/Medications		
Before:		Time:		(systolic):		Heart Rate (per min)	Type/Units	Pre	Post
After:		Time:		(diastolic):					

Lunch

	Totals:								

Blood Glucose Levels				Blood Pressure Levels			Insulin/Medications		
Before:		Time:		(systolic):		Heart Rate (per min)	Type/Units	Pre	Post
After:		Time:		(diastolic):					

Snack #2

	Totals:								

Blood Glucose Levels				Blood Pressure Levels			Insulin/Medications		
Before:		Time:		(systolic):		Heart Rate (per min)	Type/Units	Pre	Post
After:		Time:		(diastolic):					

Dinner

	Totals:								

Blood Glucose Levels				Blood Pressure Levels			Insulin/Medications		
Before:		Time:		(systolic):		Heart Rate (per min)	Type/Units	Pre	Post
After:		Time:		(diastolic):					

Fasting Blood Sugar:

_____

Water Intake:

total ounces _____

Fitness Log:

Activity	Min

Sleep Log:

Total Hours _____

Notes:

DAILY LOG
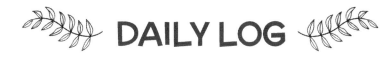

Date: ___/___/_____   **M T W Th F Sa Su**

Breakfast

Meal	Calories	Fat (g)	Carbs (g)	Sugar (g)	Fiber (g)	Net Carb (carbs-fiber)	Protein (g)	Sodium (mg)
Totals:								

Blood Glucose Levels			Blood Pressure Levels		Insulin/Medications		
Before:		Time:	(systolic):	Heart Rate (per min)	Type/Units	Pre	Post
After:		Time:	(diastolic):				

Snack #1

Totals:								

Blood Glucose Levels			Blood Pressure Levels		Insulin/Medications		
Before:		Time:	(systolic):	Heart Rate (per min)	Type/Units	Pre	Post
After:		Time:	(diastolic):				

Lunch

Totals:								

Blood Glucose Levels			Blood Pressure Levels		Insulin/Medications		
Before:		Time:	(systolic):	Heart Rate (per min)	Type/Units	Pre	Post
After:		Time:	(diastolic):				

Snack #2

Totals:								

Blood Glucose Levels			Blood Pressure Levels		Insulin/Medications		
Before:		Time:	(systolic):	Heart Rate (per min)	Type/Units	Pre	Post
After:		Time:	(diastolic):				

Dinner

Totals:								

Blood Glucose Levels			Blood Pressure Levels		Insulin/Medications		
Before:		Time:	(systolic):	Heart Rate (per min)	Type/Units	Pre	Post
After:		Time:	(diastolic):				

Fasting Blood Sugar:
_____

Water Intake:
total ounces _____

Fitness Log:

Activity	Min

Sleep Log:
Total Hours _____

Notes:
_____
_____
_____
_____
_____
_____
_____
_____
_____
_____
_____

DAILY LOG

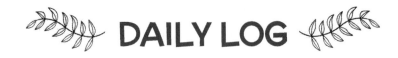

Date: ___/___/_____   **M   T   W   Th   F   Sa   Su**

	Meal	Calories	Fat (g)	Carbs (g)	Sugar (g)	Fiber (g)	Net Carb (carbs-fiber)	Protein (g)	Sodium (mg)
Breakfast									
	Totals:								

Breakfast

Blood Glucose Levels				Blood Pressure Levels		Insulin/Medications		
					Heart Rate (per min)	Type/Units	Pre	Post
Before:		Time:		(systolic):				
After:		Time:		(diastolic):				

Snack #1

	Totals:								

Blood Glucose Levels				Blood Pressure Levels		Insulin/Medications		
					Heart Rate (per min)	Type/Units	Pre	Post
Before:		Time:		(systolic):				
After:		Time:		(diastolic):				

Lunch

	Totals:								

Blood Glucose Levels				Blood Pressure Levels		Insulin/Medications		
					Heart Rate (per min)	Type/Units	Pre	Post
Before:		Time:		(systolic):				
After:		Time:		(diastolic):				

Snack #2

	Totals:								

Blood Glucose Levels				Blood Pressure Levels		Insulin/Medications		
					Heart Rate (per min)	Type/Units	Pre	Post
Before:		Time:		(systolic):				
After:		Time:		(diastolic):				

Dinner

	Totals:								

Blood Glucose Levels				Blood Pressure Levels		Insulin/Medications		
					Heart Rate (per min)	Type/Units	Pre	Post
Before:		Time:		(systolic):				
After:		Time:		(diastolic):				

Fasting Blood Sugar:

_____

Water Intake:

total ounces _____

Fitness Log:

Activity	Min

Sleep Log:

Total Hours _____

Notes:

_____
_____
_____
_____
_____
_____
_____
_____
_____

DAILY LOG

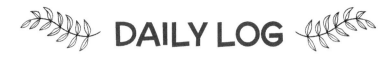

Date: ___/___/_____   M T W Th F Sa Su

Breakfast

Meal	Calories	Fat (g)	Carbs (g)	Sugar (g)	Fiber (g)	Net Carb (carbs-fiber)	Protein (g)	Sodium (mg)
Totals:								

Blood Glucose Levels			Blood Pressure Levels			Insulin/Medications		
Before:		Time:	(systolic):		Heart Rate (per min)	Type/Units	Pre	Post
After:		Time:	(diastolic):					

Snack #1

Totals:								

Blood Glucose Levels			Blood Pressure Levels			Insulin/Medications		
Before:		Time:	(systolic):		Heart Rate (per min)	Type/Units	Pre	Post
After:		Time:	(diastolic):					

Lunch

Totals:								

Blood Glucose Levels			Blood Pressure Levels			Insulin/Medications		
Before:		Time:	(systolic):		Heart Rate (per min)	Type/Units	Pre	Post
After:		Time:	(diastolic):					

Snack #2

Totals:								

Blood Glucose Levels			Blood Pressure Levels			Insulin/Medications		
Before:		Time:	(systolic):		Heart Rate (per min)	Type/Units	Pre	Post
After:		Time:	(diastolic):					

Dinner

Totals:								

Blood Glucose Levels			Blood Pressure Levels			Insulin/Medications		
Before:		Time:	(systolic):		Heart Rate (per min)	Type/Units	Pre	Post
After:		Time:	(diastolic):					

Fasting Blood Sugar:

_____

Water Intake:

total ounces _____

Fitness Log:

Activity	Min

Sleep Log:

Total Hours _____

Notes:

DAILY LOG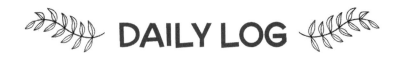

Date: ___/___/_____   **M T W Th F Sa Su**

Breakfast

Meal	Calories	Fat (g)	Carbs (g)	Sugar (g)	Fiber (g)	Net Carb (carbs-fiber)	Protein (g)	Sodium (mg)
Totals:								

Blood Glucose Levels		Blood Pressure Levels		Insulin/Medications		
Before:	Time:	(systolic):	Heart Rate (per min)	Type/Units	Pre	Post
After:	Time:	(diastolic):				

Snack #1

Totals:								

Blood Glucose Levels		Blood Pressure Levels		Insulin/Medications		
Before:	Time:	(systolic):	Heart Rate (per min)	Type/Units	Pre	Post
After:	Time:	(diastolic):				

Lunch

Totals:								

Blood Glucose Levels		Blood Pressure Levels		Insulin/Medications		
Before:	Time:	(systolic):	Heart Rate (per min)	Type/Units	Pre	Post
After:	Time:	(diastolic):				

Snack #2

Totals:								

Blood Glucose Levels		Blood Pressure Levels		Insulin/Medications		
Before:	Time:	(systolic):	Heart Rate (per min)	Type/Units	Pre	Post
After:	Time:	(diastolic):				

Dinner

Totals:								

Blood Glucose Levels		Blood Pressure Levels		Insulin/Medications		
Before:	Time:	(systolic):	Heart Rate (per min)	Type/Units	Pre	Post
After:	Time:	(diastolic):				

Fasting Blood Sugar:
_____

Water Intake:
total ounces _____

Fitness Log:
Activity	Min

Sleep Log:
Total Hours _____

Notes:
_____
_____
_____
_____
_____
_____
_____
_____
_____

DAILY LOG

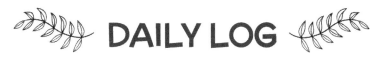

Date: ___/___/_____   **M T W Th F Sa Su**

Breakfast

	Meal	Calories	Fat (g)	Carbs (g)	Sugar (g)	Fiber (g)	Net Carb (carbs-fiber)	Protein (g)	Sodium (mg)
	Totals:								

Blood Glucose Levels				Blood Pressure Levels			Insulin/Medications		
Before:		Time:		(systolic):		Heart Rate (per min)	Type/Units	Pre	Post
After:		Time:		(diastolic):					

Snack #1

	Totals:								

Blood Glucose Levels				Blood Pressure Levels			Insulin/Medications		
Before:		Time:		(systolic):		Heart Rate (per min)	Type/Units	Pre	Post
After:		Time:		(diastolic):					

Lunch

	Totals:								

Blood Glucose Levels				Blood Pressure Levels			Insulin/Medications		
Before:		Time:		(systolic):		Heart Rate (per min)	Type/Units	Pre	Post
After:		Time:		(diastolic):					

Snack #2

	Totals:								

Blood Glucose Levels				Blood Pressure Levels			Insulin/Medications		
Before:		Time:		(systolic):		Heart Rate (per min)	Type/Units	Pre	Post
After:		Time:		(diastolic):					

Dinner

	Totals:								

Blood Glucose Levels				Blood Pressure Levels			Insulin/Medications		
Before:		Time:		(systolic):		Heart Rate (per min)	Type/Units	Pre	Post
After:		Time:		(diastolic):					

Fasting Blood Sugar:
_____

Water Intake:
total ounces _____

Fitness Log:

Activity	Min

Sleep Log:
Total Hours _____

Notes:

DAILY LOG

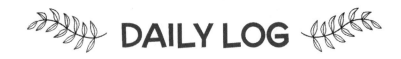

Date: ___/___/_____   **M   T   W   Th   F   Sa   Su**

Breakfast

Meal	Calories	Fat (g)	Carbs (g)	Sugar (g)	Fiber (g)	Net Carb (carbs-fiber)	Protein (g)	Sodium (mg)
Totals:								

Blood Glucose Levels		Blood Pressure Levels		Insulin/Medications		
			Heart Rate (per min)	Type/Units	Pre	Post
Before:	Time:	(systolic):				
After:	Time:	(diastolic):				

Snack #1

Totals:								

Blood Glucose Levels		Blood Pressure Levels		Insulin/Medications		
			Heart Rate (per min)	Type/Units	Pre	Post
Before:	Time:	(systolic):				
After:	Time:	(diastolic):				

Lunch

Totals:								

Blood Glucose Levels		Blood Pressure Levels		Insulin/Medications		
			Heart Rate (per min)	Type/Units	Pre	Post
Before:	Time:	(systolic):				
After:	Time:	(diastolic):				

Snack #2

Totals:								

Blood Glucose Levels		Blood Pressure Levels		Insulin/Medications		
			Heart Rate (per min)	Type/Units	Pre	Post
Before:	Time:	(systolic):				
After:	Time:	(diastolic):				

Dinner

Totals:								

Blood Glucose Levels		Blood Pressure Levels		Insulin/Medications		
			Heart Rate (per min)	Type/Units	Pre	Post
Before:	Time:	(systolic):				
After:	Time:	(diastolic):				

Fasting Blood Sugar:

_____

Water Intake:

total ounces _____

Fitness Log:

Activity	Min

Sleep Log:

Total Hours _____

Notes:

_____
_____
_____
_____
_____
_____
_____
_____

DAILY LOG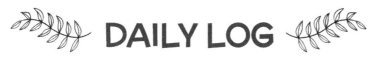

Date: ___/___/_____   **M T W Th F Sa Su**

Breakfast

Meal	Calories	Fat (g)	Carbs (g)	Sugar (g)	Fiber (g)	Net Carb (carbs-fiber)	Protein (g)	Sodium (mg)
Totals:								

Blood Glucose Levels			Blood Pressure Levels			Insulin/Medications		
Before:		Time:		(systolic):	Heart Rate (per min)	Type/Units	Pre	Post
After:		Time:		(diastolic):				

Snack #1

Totals:								

Blood Glucose Levels			Blood Pressure Levels			Insulin/Medications		
Before:		Time:		(systolic):	Heart Rate (per min)	Type/Units	Pre	Post
After:		Time:		(diastolic):				

Lunch

Totals:								

Blood Glucose Levels			Blood Pressure Levels			Insulin/Medications		
Before:		Time:		(systolic):	Heart Rate (per min)	Type/Units	Pre	Post
After:		Time:		(diastolic):				

Snack #2

Totals:								

Blood Glucose Levels			Blood Pressure Levels			Insulin/Medications		
Before:		Time:		(systolic):	Heart Rate (per min)	Type/Units	Pre	Post
After:		Time:		(diastolic):				

Dinner

Totals:								

Blood Glucose Levels			Blood Pressure Levels			Insulin/Medications		
Before:		Time:		(systolic):	Heart Rate (per min)	Type/Units	Pre	Post
After:		Time:		(diastolic):				

Fasting Blood Sugar:

_____

Water Intake:

total ounces _____

Fitness Log:

Activity	Min

Sleep Log:

Total Hours _____

Notes:

_____
_____
_____
_____
_____
_____
_____
_____
_____
_____

DAILY LOG

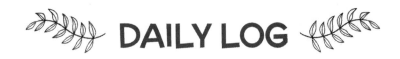

Date: ___/___/_____   **M T W Th F Sa Su**

Breakfast

	Meal		Calories	Fat (g)	Carbs (g)	Sugar (g)	Fiber (g)	Net Carb (carbs-fiber)	Protein (g)	Sodium (mg)
	Totals:									

Blood Glucose Levels				Blood Pressure Levels			Insulin/Medications		
						Heart Rate (per min)	Type/Units	Pre	Post
Before:		Time:		(systolic):					
After:		Time:		(diastolic):					

Snack #1

	Meal		Calories	Fat (g)	Carbs (g)	Sugar (g)	Fiber (g)	Net Carb (carbs-fiber)	Protein (g)	Sodium (mg)
	Totals:									

Blood Glucose Levels				Blood Pressure Levels			Insulin/Medications		
						Heart Rate (per min)	Type/Units	Pre	Post
Before:		Time:		(systolic):					
After:		Time:		(diastolic):					

Lunch

	Meal		Calories	Fat (g)	Carbs (g)	Sugar (g)	Fiber (g)	Net Carb (carbs-fiber)	Protein (g)	Sodium (mg)
	Totals:									

Blood Glucose Levels				Blood Pressure Levels			Insulin/Medications		
						Heart Rate (per min)	Type/Units	Pre	Post
Before:		Time:		(systolic):					
After:		Time:		(diastolic):					

Snack #2

	Meal		Calories	Fat (g)	Carbs (g)	Sugar (g)	Fiber (g)	Net Carb (carbs-fiber)	Protein (g)	Sodium (mg)
	Totals:									

Blood Glucose Levels				Blood Pressure Levels			Insulin/Medications		
						Heart Rate (per min)	Type/Units	Pre	Post
Before:		Time:		(systolic):					
After:		Time:		(diastolic):					

Dinner

	Meal		Calories	Fat (g)	Carbs (g)	Sugar (g)	Fiber (g)	Net Carb (carbs-fiber)	Protein (g)	Sodium (mg)
	Totals:									

Blood Glucose Levels				Blood Pressure Levels			Insulin/Medications		
						Heart Rate (per min)	Type/Units	Pre	Post
Before:		Time:		(systolic):					
After:		Time:		(diastolic):					

Fasting Blood Sugar:

_____

Water Intake:

total ounces _____

Fitness Log:

Activity	Min

Sleep Log:

Total Hours _____

Notes:

_____
_____
_____
_____
_____
_____
_____
_____

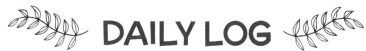

DAILY LOG

Date: ___/___/_____   **M   T   W   Th   F   Sa   Su**

Breakfast

Meal	Calories	Fat (g)	Carbs (g)	Sugar (g)	Fiber (g)	Net Carb (carbs-fiber)	Protein (g)	Sodium (mg)
Totals:								

Blood Glucose Levels			Blood Pressure Levels			Insulin/Medications		
				Heart Rate (per min)		Type/Units	Pre	Post
Before:		Time:	(systolic):					
After:		Time:	(diastolic):					

Snack #1

Totals:								

Blood Glucose Levels			Blood Pressure Levels			Insulin/Medications		
				Heart Rate (per min)		Type/Units	Pre	Post
Before:		Time:	(systolic):					
After:		Time:	(diastolic):					

Lunch

Totals:								

Blood Glucose Levels			Blood Pressure Levels			Insulin/Medications		
				Heart Rate (per min)		Type/Units	Pre	Post
Before:		Time:	(systolic):					
After:		Time:	(diastolic):					

Snack #2

Totals:								

Blood Glucose Levels			Blood Pressure Levels			Insulin/Medications		
				Heart Rate (per min)		Type/Units	Pre	Post
Before:		Time:	(systolic):					
After:		Time:	(diastolic):					

Dinner

Totals:								

Blood Glucose Levels			Blood Pressure Levels			Insulin/Medications		
				Heart Rate (per min)		Type/Units	Pre	Post
Before:		Time:	(systolic):					
After:		Time:	(diastolic):					

Fasting Blood Sugar:

_____

Water Intake:

total ounces _____

Fitness Log:

Activity	Min

Sleep Log:

Total Hours _____

Notes:

_____
_____
_____
_____
_____
_____
_____
_____
_____
_____

DAILY LOG

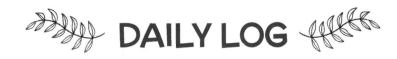

Date: ____/____/_____   **M T W Th F Sa Su**

Breakfast

	Meal	Calories	Fat (g)	Carbs (g)	Sugar (g)	Fiber (g)	Net Carb (carbs-fiber)	Protein (g)	Sodium (mg)
Totals:									

Blood Glucose Levels				Blood Pressure Levels			Insulin/Medications		
						Heart Rate (per min)	Type/Units	Pre	Post
Before:		Time:		(systolic):					
After:		Time:		(diastolic):					

Snack #1

	Meal	Calories	Fat (g)	Carbs (g)	Sugar (g)	Fiber (g)	Net Carb (carbs-fiber)	Protein (g)	Sodium (mg)
Totals:									

Blood Glucose Levels				Blood Pressure Levels			Insulin/Medications		
						Heart Rate (per min)	Type/Units	Pre	Post
Before:		Time:		(systolic):					
After:		Time:		(diastolic):					

Lunch

	Meal	Calories	Fat (g)	Carbs (g)	Sugar (g)	Fiber (g)	Net Carb (carbs-fiber)	Protein (g)	Sodium (mg)
Totals:									

Blood Glucose Levels				Blood Pressure Levels			Insulin/Medications		
						Heart Rate (per min)	Type/Units	Pre	Post
Before:		Time:		(systolic):					
After:		Time:		(diastolic):					

Snack #2

	Meal	Calories	Fat (g)	Carbs (g)	Sugar (g)	Fiber (g)	Net Carb (carbs-fiber)	Protein (g)	Sodium (mg)
Totals:									

Blood Glucose Levels				Blood Pressure Levels			Insulin/Medications		
						Heart Rate (per min)	Type/Units	Pre	Post
Before:		Time:		(systolic):					
After:		Time:		(diastolic):					

Dinner

	Meal	Calories	Fat (g)	Carbs (g)	Sugar (g)	Fiber (g)	Net Carb (carbs-fiber)	Protein (g)	Sodium (mg)
Totals:									

Blood Glucose Levels				Blood Pressure Levels			Insulin/Medications		
						Heart Rate (per min)	Type/Units	Pre	Post
Before:		Time:		(systolic):					
After:		Time:		(diastolic):					

Fasting Blood Sugar:

_____

Water Intake:

🍶 🍶 🍶 🍶 🍶 🍶 🍶 🍶

total ounces _____

Fitness Log:

Activity	Min

Sleep Log:

Total Hours _____

Notes:

_____
_____
_____
_____
_____
_____
_____
_____
_____
_____
_____
_____

DAILY LOG

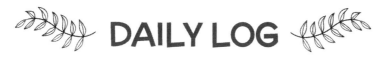

Date: ___/___/_____

M T W Th F Sa Su

Breakfast

Meal	Calories	Fat (g)	Carbs (g)	Sugar (g)	Fiber (g)	Net Carb (carbs-fiber)	Protein (g)	Sodium (mg)
Totals:								

Blood Glucose Levels				Blood Pressure Levels			Insulin/Medications		
Before:		Time:		(systolic):		Heart Rate (per min)	Type/Units	Pre	Post
After:		Time:		(diastolic):					

Snack #1

Totals:								

Blood Glucose Levels				Blood Pressure Levels			Insulin/Medications		
Before:		Time:		(systolic):		Heart Rate (per min)	Type/Units	Pre	Post
After:		Time:		(diastolic):					

Lunch

Totals:								

Blood Glucose Levels				Blood Pressure Levels			Insulin/Medications		
Before:		Time:		(systolic):		Heart Rate (per min)	Type/Units	Pre	Post
After:		Time:		(diastolic):					

Snack #2

Totals:								

Blood Glucose Levels				Blood Pressure Levels			Insulin/Medications		
Before:		Time:		(systolic):		Heart Rate (per min)	Type/Units	Pre	Post
After:		Time:		(diastolic):					

Dinner

Totals:								

Blood Glucose Levels				Blood Pressure Levels			Insulin/Medications		
Before:		Time:		(systolic):		Heart Rate (per min)	Type/Units	Pre	Post
After:		Time:		(diastolic):					

Fasting Blood Sugar:

_____

Water Intake:

total ounces _____

Fitness Log:

Activity	Min

Sleep Log:

Total Hours _____

Notes:

DAILY LOG

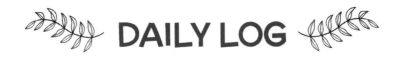

Date: ____/____/_____   **M T W Th F Sa Su**

Breakfast

	Meal	Calories	Fat (g)	Carbs (g)	Sugar (g)	Fiber (g)	Net Carb (carbs-fiber)	Protein (g)	Sodium (mg)
	Totals:								

Blood Glucose Levels				Blood Pressure Levels			Insulin/Medications		
Before:		Time:		(systolic):		Heart Rate (per min)	Type/Units	Pre	Post
After:		Time:		(diastolic):					

Snack #1

	Totals:								

Blood Glucose Levels				Blood Pressure Levels			Insulin/Medications		
Before:		Time:		(systolic):		Heart Rate (per min)	Type/Units	Pre	Post
After:		Time:		(diastolic):					

Lunch

	Totals:								

Blood Glucose Levels				Blood Pressure Levels			Insulin/Medications		
Before:		Time:		(systolic):		Heart Rate (per min)	Type/Units	Pre	Post
After:		Time:		(diastolic):					

Snack #2

	Totals:								

Blood Glucose Levels				Blood Pressure Levels			Insulin/Medications		
Before:		Time:		(systolic):		Heart Rate (per min)	Type/Units	Pre	Post
After:		Time:		(diastolic):					

Dinner

	Totals:								

Blood Glucose Levels				Blood Pressure Levels			Insulin/Medications		
Before:		Time:		(systolic):		Heart Rate (per min)	Type/Units	Pre	Post
After:		Time:		(diastolic):					

Fasting Blood Sugar:

_____

Water Intake:

total ounces _____

Fitness Log:

Activity	Min

Sleep Log:

Total Hours _____

Notes:

_____
_____
_____
_____
_____
_____
_____
_____
_____
_____
_____
_____

DAILY LOG

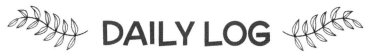

Date: ___/___/_____   **M T W Th F Sa Su**

Breakfast

	Meal	Calories	Fat (g)	Carbs (g)	Sugar (g)	Fiber (g)	Net Carb (carbs-fiber)	Protein (g)	Sodium (mg)
	Totals:								

Blood Glucose Levels				Blood Pressure Levels			Insulin/Medications		
Before:		Time:		(systolic):		Heart Rate (per min)	Type/Units	Pre	Post
After:		Time:		(diastolic):					

Snack #1

	Totals:								

Blood Glucose Levels				Blood Pressure Levels			Insulin/Medications		
Before:		Time:		(systolic):		Heart Rate (per min)	Type/Units	Pre	Post
After:		Time:		(diastolic):					

Lunch

	Totals:								

Blood Glucose Levels				Blood Pressure Levels			Insulin/Medications		
Before:		Time:		(systolic):		Heart Rate (per min)	Type/Units	Pre	Post
After:		Time:		(diastolic):					

Snack #2

	Totals:								

Blood Glucose Levels				Blood Pressure Levels			Insulin/Medications		
Before:		Time:		(systolic):		Heart Rate (per min)	Type/Units	Pre	Post
After:		Time:		(diastolic):					

Dinner

	Totals:								

Blood Glucose Levels				Blood Pressure Levels			Insulin/Medications		
Before:		Time:		(systolic):		Heart Rate (per min)	Type/Units	Pre	Post
After:		Time:		(diastolic):					

Fasting Blood Sugar:

_____

Water Intake:

total ounces _____

Fitness Log:

Activity	Min

Sleep Log:

Total Hours _____

Notes:

_____
_____
_____
_____
_____
_____
_____
_____
_____

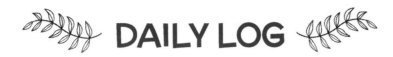

DAILY LOG

Date: ____/____/_____   M   T   W   Th   F   Sa   Su

Breakfast

Meal	Calories	Fat (g)	Carbs (g)	Sugar (g)	Fiber (g)	Net Carb (carbs-fiber)	Protein (g)	Sodium (mg)
Totals:								

Blood Glucose Levels			Blood Pressure Levels		Insulin/Medications		
				Heart Rate (per min)	Type/Units	Pre	Post
Before:		Time:	(systolic):				
After:		Time:	(diastolic):				

Snack #1

Meal	Calories	Fat (g)	Carbs (g)	Sugar (g)	Fiber (g)	Net Carb (carbs-fiber)	Protein (g)	Sodium (mg)
Totals:								

Blood Glucose Levels			Blood Pressure Levels		Insulin/Medications		
				Heart Rate (per min)	Type/Units	Pre	Post
Before:		Time:	(systolic):				
After:		Time:	(diastolic):				

Lunch

Meal	Calories	Fat (g)	Carbs (g)	Sugar (g)	Fiber (g)	Net Carb (carbs-fiber)	Protein (g)	Sodium (mg)
Totals:								

Blood Glucose Levels			Blood Pressure Levels		Insulin/Medications		
				Heart Rate (per min)	Type/Units	Pre	Post
Before:		Time:	(systolic):				
After:		Time:	(diastolic):				

Snack #2

Meal	Calories	Fat (g)	Carbs (g)	Sugar (g)	Fiber (g)	Net Carb (carbs-fiber)	Protein (g)	Sodium (mg)
Totals:								

Blood Glucose Levels			Blood Pressure Levels		Insulin/Medications		
				Heart Rate (per min)	Type/Units	Pre	Post
Before:		Time:	(systolic):				
After:		Time:	(diastolic):				

Dinner

Meal	Calories	Fat (g)	Carbs (g)	Sugar (g)	Fiber (g)	Net Carb (carbs-fiber)	Protein (g)	Sodium (mg)
Totals:								

Blood Glucose Levels			Blood Pressure Levels		Insulin/Medications		
				Heart Rate (per min)	Type/Units	Pre	Post
Before:		Time:	(systolic):				
After:		Time:	(diastolic):				

Fasting Blood Sugar:

_____

Water Intake:

total ounces _____

Fitness Log:

Activity	Min

Sleep Log:

Total Hours _____

Notes:

_____
_____
_____
_____
_____
_____
_____
_____
_____
_____
_____

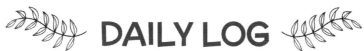

DAILY LOG

Date: ___/___/_____   M   T   W   Th   F   Sa   Su

Breakfast

Meal	Calories	Fat (g)	Carbs (g)	Sugar (g)	Fiber (g)	Net Carb (carbs-fiber)	Protein (g)	Sodium (mg)
Totals:								

Blood Glucose Levels			Blood Pressure Levels			Insulin/Medications		
Before:		Time:	(systolic):		Heart Rate (per min)	Type/Units	Pre	Post
After:		Time:	(diastolic):					

Snack #1

Totals:								

Blood Glucose Levels			Blood Pressure Levels			Insulin/Medications		
Before:		Time:	(systolic):		Heart Rate (per min)	Type/Units	Pre	Post
After:		Time:	(diastolic):					

Lunch

Totals:								

Blood Glucose Levels			Blood Pressure Levels			Insulin/Medications		
Before:		Time:	(systolic):		Heart Rate (per min)	Type/Units	Pre	Post
After:		Time:	(diastolic):					

Snack #2

Totals:								

Blood Glucose Levels			Blood Pressure Levels			Insulin/Medications		
Before:		Time:	(systolic):		Heart Rate (per min)	Type/Units	Pre	Post
After:		Time:	(diastolic):					

Dinner

Totals:								

Blood Glucose Levels			Blood Pressure Levels			Insulin/Medications		
Before:		Time:	(systolic):		Heart Rate (per min)	Type/Units	Pre	Post
After:		Time:	(diastolic):					

Fasting Blood Sugar:

_____

Water Intake:

total ounces _____

Fitness Log:

Activity	Min

Sleep Log:

Total Hours _____

Notes:

_____
_____
_____
_____
_____
_____
_____
_____
_____
_____
_____

DAILY LOG

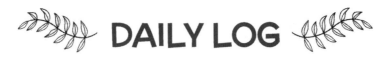

Date: ___/___/_____   M T W Th F Sa Su

Breakfast

Meal	Calories	Fat (g)	Carbs (g)	Sugar (g)	Fiber (g)	Net Carb (carbs-fiber)	Protein (g)	Sodium (mg)
Totals:								

Blood Glucose Levels			Blood Pressure Levels			Insulin/Medications		
Before:		Time:	(systolic):		Heart Rate (per min)	Type/Units	Pre	Post
After:		Time:	(diastolic):					

Snack #1

Meal	Calories	Fat (g)	Carbs (g)	Sugar (g)	Fiber (g)	Net Carb (carbs-fiber)	Protein (g)	Sodium (mg)
Totals:								

Blood Glucose Levels			Blood Pressure Levels			Insulin/Medications		
Before:		Time:	(systolic):		Heart Rate (per min)	Type/Units	Pre	Post
After:		Time:	(diastolic):					

Lunch

Meal	Calories	Fat (g)	Carbs (g)	Sugar (g)	Fiber (g)	Net Carb (carbs-fiber)	Protein (g)	Sodium (mg)
Totals:								

Blood Glucose Levels			Blood Pressure Levels			Insulin/Medications		
Before:		Time:	(systolic):		Heart Rate (per min)	Type/Units	Pre	Post
After:		Time:	(diastolic):					

Snack #2

Meal	Calories	Fat (g)	Carbs (g)	Sugar (g)	Fiber (g)	Net Carb (carbs-fiber)	Protein (g)	Sodium (mg)
Totals:								

Blood Glucose Levels			Blood Pressure Levels			Insulin/Medications		
Before:		Time:	(systolic):		Heart Rate (per min)	Type/Units	Pre	Post
After:		Time:	(diastolic):					

Dinner

Meal	Calories	Fat (g)	Carbs (g)	Sugar (g)	Fiber (g)	Net Carb (carbs-fiber)	Protein (g)	Sodium (mg)
Totals:								

Blood Glucose Levels			Blood Pressure Levels			Insulin/Medications		
Before:		Time:	(systolic):		Heart Rate (per min)	Type/Units	Pre	Post
After:		Time:	(diastolic):					

Fasting Blood Sugar:

_____

Water Intake:

total ounces _____

Fitness Log:

Activity	Min

Sleep Log:

Total Hours _____

Notes:

_____
_____
_____
_____
_____
_____
_____
_____
_____
_____
_____

DAILY LOG

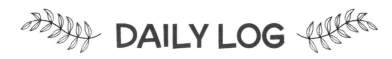

Date: ___/___/_____   **M T W Th F Sa Su**

Breakfast

Meal	Calories	Fat (g)	Carbs (g)	Sugar (g)	Fiber (g)	Net Carb (carbs-fiber)	Protein (g)	Sodium (mg)
Totals:								

Blood Glucose Levels			Blood Pressure Levels		Insulin/Medications		
Before:		Time:		(systolic):	Heart Rate (per min)	Type/Units	Pre	Post
After:		Time:		(diastolic):				

Snack #1

Totals:								

Blood Glucose Levels			Blood Pressure Levels		Insulin/Medications		
Before:		Time:		(systolic):	Heart Rate (per min)	Type/Units	Pre	Post
After:		Time:		(diastolic):				

Lunch

Totals:								

Blood Glucose Levels			Blood Pressure Levels		Insulin/Medications		
Before:		Time:		(systolic):	Heart Rate (per min)	Type/Units	Pre	Post
After:		Time:		(diastolic):				

Snack #2

Totals:								

Blood Glucose Levels			Blood Pressure Levels		Insulin/Medications		
Before:		Time:		(systolic):	Heart Rate (per min)	Type/Units	Pre	Post
After:		Time:		(diastolic):				

Dinner

Totals:								

Blood Glucose Levels			Blood Pressure Levels		Insulin/Medications		
Before:		Time:		(systolic):	Heart Rate (per min)	Type/Units	Pre	Post
After:		Time:		(diastolic):				

Fasting Blood Sugar:
_____

Water Intake:
total ounces _____

Fitness Log:

Activity	Min

Sleep Log:
Total Hours _____

Notes:
_____
_____
_____
_____
_____
_____
_____
_____
_____
_____

DAILY LOG

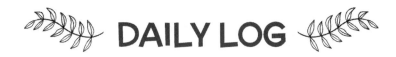

Date: ___/___/_____   **M T W Th F Sa Su**

Breakfast

Meal	Calories	Fat (g)	Carbs (g)	Sugar (g)	Fiber (g)	Net Carb (carbs-fiber)	Protein (g)	Sodium (mg)
Totals:								

Blood Glucose Levels				Blood Pressure Levels			Insulin/Medications		
Before:		Time:		(systolic):		Heart Rate (per min)	Type/Units	Pre	Post
After:		Time:		(diastolic):					

Snack #1

Totals:								

Blood Glucose Levels				Blood Pressure Levels			Insulin/Medications		
Before:		Time:		(systolic):		Heart Rate (per min)	Type/Units	Pre	Post
After:		Time:		(diastolic):					

Lunch

Totals:								

Blood Glucose Levels				Blood Pressure Levels			Insulin/Medications		
Before:		Time:		(systolic):		Heart Rate (per min)	Type/Units	Pre	Post
After:		Time:		(diastolic):					

Snack #2

Totals:								

Blood Glucose Levels				Blood Pressure Levels			Insulin/Medications		
Before:		Time:		(systolic):		Heart Rate (per min)	Type/Units	Pre	Post
After:		Time:		(diastolic):					

Dinner

Totals:								

Blood Glucose Levels				Blood Pressure Levels			Insulin/Medications		
Before:		Time:		(systolic):		Heart Rate (per min)	Type/Units	Pre	Post
After:		Time:		(diastolic):					

Fasting Blood Sugar:

_____

Water Intake:

total ounces _____

Fitness Log:

Activity	Min

Sleep Log:

Total Hours _____

Notes:

DAILY LOG

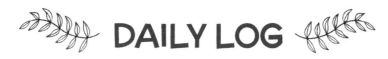

Date: ___/___/_____   **M T W Th F Sa Su**

Breakfast

Meal	Calories	Fat (g)	Carbs (g)	Sugar (g)	Fiber (g)	Net Carb (carbs-fiber)	Protein (g)	Sodium (mg)
Totals:								

Blood Glucose Levels			Blood Pressure Levels		Insulin/Medications		
Before:		Time:	(systolic):	Heart Rate (per min)	Type/Units	Pre	Post
After:		Time:	(diastolic):				

Snack #1

Totals:								

Blood Glucose Levels			Blood Pressure Levels		Insulin/Medications		
Before:		Time:	(systolic):	Heart Rate (per min)	Type/Units	Pre	Post
After:		Time:	(diastolic):				

Lunch

Totals:								

Blood Glucose Levels			Blood Pressure Levels		Insulin/Medications		
Before:		Time:	(systolic):	Heart Rate (per min)	Type/Units	Pre	Post
After:		Time:	(diastolic):				

Snack #2

Totals:								

Blood Glucose Levels			Blood Pressure Levels		Insulin/Medications		
Before:		Time:	(systolic):	Heart Rate (per min)	Type/Units	Pre	Post
After:		Time:	(diastolic):				

Dinner

Totals:								

Blood Glucose Levels			Blood Pressure Levels		Insulin/Medications		
Before:		Time:	(systolic):	Heart Rate (per min)	Type/Units	Pre	Post
After:		Time:	(diastolic):				

Fasting Blood Sugar:

_____

Water Intake:

total ounces _____

Fitness Log:

Activity	Min

Sleep Log:

Total Hours _____

Notes:

DAILY LOG

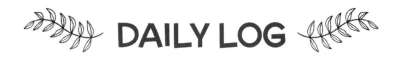

Date: ___/___/_____   **M T W Th F Sa Su**

Breakfast

	Meal	Calories	Fat (g)	Carbs (g)	Sugar (g)	Fiber (g)	Net Carb (carbs-fiber)	Protein (g)	Sodium (mg)
	Totals:								

Blood Glucose Levels				Blood Pressure Levels			Insulin/Medications		
Before:		Time:		(systolic):		Heart Rate (per min)	Type/Units	Pre	Post
After:		Time:		(diastolic):					

Snack #1

	Totals:								

Blood Glucose Levels				Blood Pressure Levels			Insulin/Medications		
Before:		Time:		(systolic):		Heart Rate (per min)	Type/Units	Pre	Post
After:		Time:		(diastolic):					

Lunch

	Totals:								

Blood Glucose Levels				Blood Pressure Levels			Insulin/Medications		
Before:		Time:		(systolic):		Heart Rate (per min)	Type/Units	Pre	Post
After:		Time:		(diastolic):					

Snack #2

	Totals:								

Blood Glucose Levels				Blood Pressure Levels			Insulin/Medications		
Before:		Time:		(systolic):		Heart Rate (per min)	Type/Units	Pre	Post
After:		Time:		(diastolic):					

Dinner

	Totals:								

Blood Glucose Levels				Blood Pressure Levels			Insulin/Medications		
Before:		Time:		(systolic):		Heart Rate (per min)	Type/Units	Pre	Post
After:		Time:		(diastolic):					

Fasting Blood Sugar:

_____

Water Intake:

total ounces _____

Fitness Log:

Activity   Min

Sleep Log:

Total Hours _____

Notes:

DAILY LOG

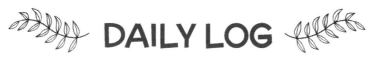

Date: ___/___/_____   M T W Th F Sa Su

Breakfast

	Meal	Calories	Fat (g)	Carbs (g)	Sugar (g)	Fiber (g)	Net Carb (carbs-fiber)	Protein (g)	Sodium (mg)
	Totals:								

Blood Glucose Levels			Blood Pressure Levels		Insulin/Medications		
Before:		Time:	(systolic):	Heart Rate (per min)	Type/Units	Pre	Post
After:		Time:	(diastolic):				

Snack #1

	Totals:								

Blood Glucose Levels			Blood Pressure Levels		Insulin/Medications		
Before:		Time:	(systolic):	Heart Rate (per min)	Type/Units	Pre	Post
After:		Time:	(diastolic):				

Lunch

	Totals:								

Blood Glucose Levels			Blood Pressure Levels		Insulin/Medications		
Before:		Time:	(systolic):	Heart Rate (per min)	Type/Units	Pre	Post
After:		Time:	(diastolic):				

Snack #2

	Totals:								

Blood Glucose Levels			Blood Pressure Levels		Insulin/Medications		
Before:		Time:	(systolic):	Heart Rate (per min)	Type/Units	Pre	Post
After:		Time:	(diastolic):				

Dinner

	Totals:								

Blood Glucose Levels			Blood Pressure Levels		Insulin/Medications		
Before:		Time:	(systolic):	Heart Rate (per min)	Type/Units	Pre	Post
After:		Time:	(diastolic):				

Fasting Blood Sugar:

_____

Water Intake:

total ounces _____

Fitness Log:

Activity	Min

Sleep Log:

Total Hours _____

Notes:

_____
_____
_____
_____
_____
_____
_____
_____
_____

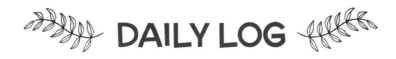

DAILY LOG

Date: ___/___/_____   **M T W Th F Sa Su**

Breakfast

Meal	Calories	Fat (g)	Carbs (g)	Sugar (g)	Fiber (g)	Net Carb (carbs-fiber)	Protein (g)	Sodium (mg)
Totals:								

Blood Glucose Levels		Blood Pressure Levels		Insulin/Medications		
Before:	Time:	(systolic):	Heart Rate (per min)	Type/Units	Pre	Post
After:	Time:	(diastolic):				

Snack #1

Totals:								

Blood Glucose Levels		Blood Pressure Levels		Insulin/Medications		
Before:	Time:	(systolic):	Heart Rate (per min)	Type/Units	Pre	Post
After:	Time:	(diastolic):				

Lunch

Totals:								

Blood Glucose Levels		Blood Pressure Levels		Insulin/Medications		
Before:	Time:	(systolic):	Heart Rate (per min)	Type/Units	Pre	Post
After:	Time:	(diastolic):				

Snack #2

Totals:								

Blood Glucose Levels		Blood Pressure Levels		Insulin/Medications		
Before:	Time:	(systolic):	Heart Rate (per min)	Type/Units	Pre	Post
After:	Time:	(diastolic):				

Dinner

Totals:								

Blood Glucose Levels		Blood Pressure Levels		Insulin/Medications		
Before:	Time:	(systolic):	Heart Rate (per min)	Type/Units	Pre	Post
After:	Time:	(diastolic):				

Fasting Blood Sugar:

_____

Water Intake:

total ounces _____

Fitness Log:

Activity	Min

Sleep Log:

Total Hours _____

Notes:

_____
_____
_____
_____
_____
_____
_____
_____
_____

DAILY LOG

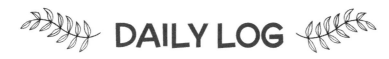

Date: ___/___/_____   **M T W Th F Sa Su**

Breakfast

	Meal	Calories	Fat (g)	Carbs (g)	Sugar (g)	Fiber (g)	Net Carb (carbs-fiber)	Protein (g)	Sodium (mg)
	Totals:								

Blood Glucose Levels			Blood Pressure Levels			Insulin/Medications		
Before:		Time:	(systolic):		Heart Rate (per min)	Type/Units	Pre	Post
After:		Time:	(diastolic):					

Snack #1

	Totals:								

Blood Glucose Levels			Blood Pressure Levels			Insulin/Medications		
Before:		Time:	(systolic):		Heart Rate (per min)	Type/Units	Pre	Post
After:		Time:	(diastolic):					

Lunch

	Totals:								

Blood Glucose Levels			Blood Pressure Levels			Insulin/Medications		
Before:		Time:	(systolic):		Heart Rate (per min)	Type/Units	Pre	Post
After:		Time:	(diastolic):					

Snack #2

	Totals:								

Blood Glucose Levels			Blood Pressure Levels			Insulin/Medications		
Before:		Time:	(systolic):		Heart Rate (per min)	Type/Units	Pre	Post
After:		Time:	(diastolic):					

Dinner

	Totals:								

Blood Glucose Levels			Blood Pressure Levels			Insulin/Medications		
Before:		Time:	(systolic):		Heart Rate (per min)	Type/Units	Pre	Post
After:		Time:	(diastolic):					

Fasting Blood Sugar:

_____

Water Intake:

total ounces _____

Fitness Log:

Activity	Min

Sleep Log:

Total Hours _____

Notes:

_____
_____
_____
_____
_____
_____
_____
_____
_____
_____

DAILY LOG

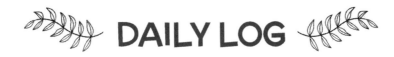

Date: ___/___/_____   **M T W Th F Sa Su**

Breakfast

	Meal	Calories	Fat (g)	Carbs (g)	Sugar (g)	Fiber (g)	Net Carb (carbs-fiber)	Protein (g)	Sodium (mg)
	Totals:								

Blood Glucose Levels				Blood Pressure Levels			Insulin/Medications		
Before:		Time:		(systolic):		Heart Rate (per min)	Type/Units	Pre	Post
After:		Time:		(diastolic):					

Snack #1

	Totals:								

Blood Glucose Levels				Blood Pressure Levels			Insulin/Medications		
Before:		Time:		(systolic):		Heart Rate (per min)	Type/Units	Pre	Post
After:		Time:		(diastolic):					

Lunch

	Totals:								

Blood Glucose Levels				Blood Pressure Levels			Insulin/Medications		
Before:		Time:		(systolic):		Heart Rate (per min)	Type/Units	Pre	Post
After:		Time:		(diastolic):					

Snack #2

	Totals:								

Blood Glucose Levels				Blood Pressure Levels			Insulin/Medications		
Before:		Time:		(systolic):		Heart Rate (per min)	Type/Units	Pre	Post
After:		Time:		(diastolic):					

Dinner

	Totals:								

Blood Glucose Levels				Blood Pressure Levels			Insulin/Medications		
Before:		Time:		(systolic):		Heart Rate (per min)	Type/Units	Pre	Post
After:		Time:		(diastolic):					

Fasting Blood Sugar:

_____

Water Intake:

total ounces _____

Fitness Log:

Activity	Min

Sleep Log:

Total Hours _____

Notes:

_____
_____
_____
_____
_____
_____
_____

DAILY LOG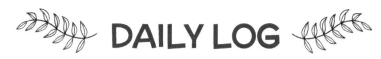

Date: ___/___/_____   **M   T   W   Th   F   Sa   Su**

Breakfast

Meal	Calories	Fat (g)	Carbs (g)	Sugar (g)	Fiber (g)	Net Carb (carbs-fiber)	Protein (g)	Sodium (mg)
Totals:								

Blood Glucose Levels				Blood Pressure Levels		Insulin/Medications		
Before:		Time:		(systolic):	Heart Rate (per min)	Type/Units	Pre	Post
After:		Time:		(diastolic):				

Snack #1

Totals:								

Blood Glucose Levels				Blood Pressure Levels		Insulin/Medications		
Before:		Time:		(systolic):	Heart Rate (per min)	Type/Units	Pre	Post
After:		Time:		(diastolic):				

Lunch

Totals:								

Blood Glucose Levels				Blood Pressure Levels		Insulin/Medications		
Before:		Time:		(systolic):	Heart Rate (per min)	Type/Units	Pre	Post
After:		Time:		(diastolic):				

Snack #2

Totals:								

Blood Glucose Levels				Blood Pressure Levels		Insulin/Medications		
Before:		Time:		(systolic):	Heart Rate (per min)	Type/Units	Pre	Post
After:		Time:		(diastolic):				

Dinner

Totals:								

Blood Glucose Levels				Blood Pressure Levels		Insulin/Medications		
Before:		Time:		(systolic):	Heart Rate (per min)	Type/Units	Pre	Post
After:		Time:		(diastolic):				

Fasting Blood Sugar:

_____

Water Intake:

total ounces _____

Fitness Log:

Activity	Min

Sleep Log:

Total Hours _____

Notes:

_____
_____
_____
_____
_____
_____
_____
_____
_____
_____

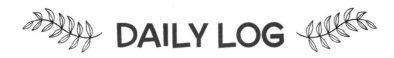

DAILY LOG

Date: ___/___/_____   **M   T   W   Th   F   Sa   Su**

Breakfast

Meal	Calories	Fat (g)	Carbs (g)	Sugar (g)	Fiber (g)	Net Carb (carbs-fiber)	Protein (g)	Sodium (mg)
Totals:								

Blood Glucose Levels				Blood Pressure Levels			Insulin/Medications		
Before:		Time:		(systolic):		Heart Rate (per min)	Type/Units	Pre	Post
After:		Time:		(diastolic):					

Snack #1

Totals:								

Blood Glucose Levels				Blood Pressure Levels			Insulin/Medications		
Before:		Time:		(systolic):		Heart Rate (per min)	Type/Units	Pre	Post
After:		Time:		(diastolic):					

Lunch

Totals:								

Blood Glucose Levels				Blood Pressure Levels			Insulin/Medications		
Before:		Time:		(systolic):		Heart Rate (per min)	Type/Units	Pre	Post
After:		Time:		(diastolic):					

Snack #2

Totals:								

Blood Glucose Levels				Blood Pressure Levels			Insulin/Medications		
Before:		Time:		(systolic):		Heart Rate (per min)	Type/Units	Pre	Post
After:		Time:		(diastolic):					

Dinner

Totals:								

Blood Glucose Levels				Blood Pressure Levels			Insulin/Medications		
Before:		Time:		(systolic):		Heart Rate (per min)	Type/Units	Pre	Post
After:		Time:		(diastolic):					

Fasting Blood Sugar:

_____

Water Intake:

total ounces _____

Fitness Log:

Activity	Min

Sleep Log:

Total Hours _____

Notes:

_____
_____
_____
_____
_____
_____
_____
_____
_____
_____

DAILY LOG

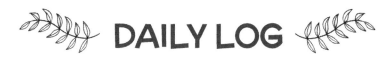

Date: ___/___/_____   **M T W Th F Sa Su**

Breakfast

	Meal	Calories	Fat (g)	Carbs (g)	Sugar (g)	Fiber (g)	Net Carb (carbs-fiber)	Protein (g)	Sodium (mg)
	Totals:								

Blood Glucose Levels			Blood Pressure Levels			Insulin/Medications		
					Heart Rate (per min)	Type/Units	Pre	Post
Before:		Time:	(systolic):					
After:		Time:	(diastolic):					

Snack #1

	Totals:								

Blood Glucose Levels			Blood Pressure Levels			Insulin/Medications		
					Heart Rate (per min)	Type/Units	Pre	Post
Before:		Time:	(systolic):					
After:		Time:	(diastolic):					

Lunch

	Totals:								

Blood Glucose Levels			Blood Pressure Levels			Insulin/Medications		
					Heart Rate (per min)	Type/Units	Pre	Post
Before:		Time:	(systolic):					
After:		Time:	(diastolic):					

Snack #2

	Totals:								

Blood Glucose Levels			Blood Pressure Levels			Insulin/Medications		
					Heart Rate (per min)	Type/Units	Pre	Post
Before:		Time:	(systolic):					
After:		Time:	(diastolic):					

Dinner

	Totals:								

Blood Glucose Levels			Blood Pressure Levels			Insulin/Medications		
					Heart Rate (per min)	Type/Units	Pre	Post
Before:		Time:	(systolic):					
After:		Time:	(diastolic):					

Fasting Blood Sugar:

_____

Water Intake:

total ounces _____

Fitness Log:

Activity	Min

Sleep Log:

Total Hours _____

Notes:

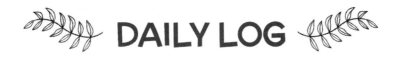

DAILY LOG

Date: ___/___/_____   **M T W Th F Sa Su**

Breakfast

Meal	Calories	Fat (g)	Carbs (g)	Sugar (g)	Fiber (g)	Net Carb (carbs-fiber)	Protein (g)	Sodium (mg)
Totals:								

Blood Glucose Levels			Blood Pressure Levels			Insulin/Medications		
Before:		Time:		(systolic):		Type/Units	Pre	Post
After:		Time:		(diastolic):	Heart Rate (per min)			

Snack #1

Totals:								

Blood Glucose Levels			Blood Pressure Levels			Insulin/Medications		
Before:		Time:		(systolic):		Type/Units	Pre	Post
After:		Time:		(diastolic):	Heart Rate (per min)			

Lunch

Totals:								

Blood Glucose Levels			Blood Pressure Levels			Insulin/Medications		
Before:		Time:		(systolic):		Type/Units	Pre	Post
After:		Time:		(diastolic):	Heart Rate (per min)			

Snack #2

Totals:								

Blood Glucose Levels			Blood Pressure Levels			Insulin/Medications		
Before:		Time:		(systolic):		Type/Units	Pre	Post
After:		Time:		(diastolic):	Heart Rate (per min)			

Dinner

Totals:								

Blood Glucose Levels			Blood Pressure Levels			Insulin/Medications		
Before:		Time:		(systolic):		Type/Units	Pre	Post
After:		Time:		(diastolic):	Heart Rate (per min)			

Fasting Blood Sugar:

_____

Water Intake:

total ounces _____

Fitness Log:

Activity	Min

Sleep Log:

Total Hours _____

Notes:

_____
_____
_____
_____
_____
_____
_____
_____
_____
_____
_____
_____

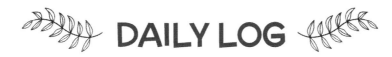

DAILY LOG

Date: ___/___/_____   **M T W Th F Sa Su**

Breakfast

	Meal	Calories	Fat (g)	Carbs (g)	Sugar (g)	Fiber (g)	Net Carb (carbs-fiber)	Protein (g)	Sodium (mg)
	Totals:								

Blood Glucose Levels			Blood Pressure Levels		Insulin/Medications		
Before:		Time:	(systolic):	Heart Rate (per min)	Type/Units	Pre	Post
After:		Time:	(diastolic):				

Snack #1

	Totals:								

Blood Glucose Levels			Blood Pressure Levels		Insulin/Medications		
Before:		Time:	(systolic):	Heart Rate (per min)	Type/Units	Pre	Post
After:		Time:	(diastolic):				

Lunch

	Totals:								

Blood Glucose Levels			Blood Pressure Levels		Insulin/Medications		
Before:		Time:	(systolic):	Heart Rate (per min)	Type/Units	Pre	Post
After:		Time:	(diastolic):				

Snack #2

	Totals:								

Blood Glucose Levels			Blood Pressure Levels		Insulin/Medications		
Before:		Time:	(systolic):	Heart Rate (per min)	Type/Units	Pre	Post
After:		Time:	(diastolic):				

Dinner

	Totals:								

Blood Glucose Levels			Blood Pressure Levels		Insulin/Medications		
Before:		Time:	(systolic):	Heart Rate (per min)	Type/Units	Pre	Post
After:		Time:	(diastolic):				

Fasting Blood Sugar:
_____

Water Intake:
total ounces _____

Fitness Log:

Activity	Min

Sleep Log:
Total Hours _____

Notes:
_____
_____
_____
_____
_____
_____
_____
_____

DAILY LOG

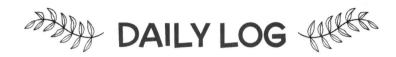

Date: ___/___/_____   **M T W Th F Sa Su**

Breakfast

Meal	Calories	Fat (g)	Carbs (g)	Sugar (g)	Fiber (g)	Net Carb (carbs-fiber)	Protein (g)	Sodium (mg)
Totals:								

Blood Glucose Levels				Blood Pressure Levels			Insulin/Medications		
Before:		Time:		(systolic):		Heart Rate (per min)	Type/Units	Pre	Post
After:		Time:		(diastolic):					

Snack #1

Totals:								

Blood Glucose Levels				Blood Pressure Levels			Insulin/Medications		
Before:		Time:		(systolic):		Heart Rate (per min)	Type/Units	Pre	Post
After:		Time:		(diastolic):					

Lunch

Totals:								

Blood Glucose Levels				Blood Pressure Levels			Insulin/Medications		
Before:		Time:		(systolic):		Heart Rate (per min)	Type/Units	Pre	Post
After:		Time:		(diastolic):					

Snack #2

Totals:								

Blood Glucose Levels				Blood Pressure Levels			Insulin/Medications		
Before:		Time:		(systolic):		Heart Rate (per min)	Type/Units	Pre	Post
After:		Time:		(diastolic):					

Dinner

Totals:								

Blood Glucose Levels				Blood Pressure Levels			Insulin/Medications		
Before:		Time:		(systolic):		Heart Rate (per min)	Type/Units	Pre	Post
After:		Time:		(diastolic):					

Fasting Blood Sugar:

_____

Water Intake:

total ounces _____

Fitness Log:

Activity	Min

Sleep Log:

Total Hours _____

Notes:

DAILY LOG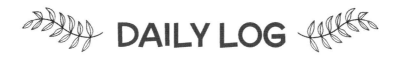

Date: ____/____/_____   **M T W Th F Sa Su**

Breakfast

	Meal	Calories	Fat (g)	Carbs (g)	Sugar (g)	Fiber (g)	Net Carb (carbs-fiber)	Protein (g)	Sodium (mg)
	Totals:								

Blood Glucose Levels				Blood Pressure Levels			Insulin/Medications		
Before:		Time:		(systolic):		Heart Rate (per min)	Type/Units	Pre	Post
After:		Time:		(diastolic):					

Snack #1

	Totals:								

Blood Glucose Levels				Blood Pressure Levels			Insulin/Medications		
Before:		Time:		(systolic):		Heart Rate (per min)	Type/Units	Pre	Post
After:		Time:		(diastolic):					

Lunch

	Totals:								

Blood Glucose Levels				Blood Pressure Levels			Insulin/Medications		
Before:		Time:		(systolic):		Heart Rate (per min)	Type/Units	Pre	Post
After:		Time:		(diastolic):					

Snack #2

	Totals:								

Blood Glucose Levels				Blood Pressure Levels			Insulin/Medications		
Before:		Time:		(systolic):		Heart Rate (per min)	Type/Units	Pre	Post
After:		Time:		(diastolic):					

Dinner

	Totals:								

Blood Glucose Levels				Blood Pressure Levels			Insulin/Medications		
Before:		Time:		(systolic):		Heart Rate (per min)	Type/Units	Pre	Post
After:		Time:		(diastolic):					

Fasting Blood Sugar:

_____

Water Intake:

total ounces _____

Fitness Log:

Activity   Min

Sleep Log:

Total Hours _____

Notes:

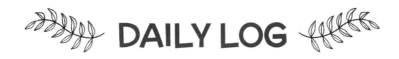

DAILY LOG

Date: ___/___/_____   **M T W Th F Sa Su**

	Meal	Calories	Fat (g)	Carbs (g)	Sugar (g)	Fiber (g)	Net Carb (carbs-fiber)	Protein (g)	Sodium (mg)
Breakfast									
	Totals:								

Breakfast

Blood Glucose Levels				Blood Pressure Levels			Insulin/Medications		
Before:		Time:		(systolic):		Heart Rate (per min)	Type/Units	Pre	Post
After:		Time:		(diastolic):					

Snack #1

	Totals:								

Blood Glucose Levels				Blood Pressure Levels			Insulin/Medications		
Before:		Time:		(systolic):		Heart Rate (per min)	Type/Units	Pre	Post
After:		Time:		(diastolic):					

Lunch

	Totals:								

Blood Glucose Levels				Blood Pressure Levels			Insulin/Medications		
Before:		Time:		(systolic):		Heart Rate (per min)	Type/Units	Pre	Post
After:		Time:		(diastolic):					

Snack #2

	Totals:								

Blood Glucose Levels				Blood Pressure Levels			Insulin/Medications		
Before:		Time:		(systolic):		Heart Rate (per min)	Type/Units	Pre	Post
After:		Time:		(diastolic):					

Dinner

	Totals:								

Blood Glucose Levels				Blood Pressure Levels			Insulin/Medications		
Before:		Time:		(systolic):		Heart Rate (per min)	Type/Units	Pre	Post
After:		Time:		(diastolic):					

Fasting Blood Sugar:

_____

Water Intake:

total ounces _____

Fitness Log:

Activity	Min

Sleep Log:

Total Hours _____

Notes:

_____
_____
_____
_____
_____
_____
_____
_____
_____
_____

DAILY LOG

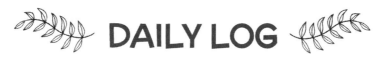

Date: ___/___/_____   **M T W Th F Sa Su**

Breakfast

Meal	Calories	Fat (g)	Carbs (g)	Sugar (g)	Fiber (g)	Net Carb (carbs-fiber)	Protein (g)	Sodium (mg)
Totals:								

Blood Glucose Levels			Blood Pressure Levels			Insulin/Medications		
Before:		Time:		(systolic):		Heart Rate (per min)	Type/Units	Pre	Post
After:		Time:		(diastolic):				

Snack #1

Meal	Calories	Fat (g)	Carbs (g)	Sugar (g)	Fiber (g)	Net Carb (carbs-fiber)	Protein (g)	Sodium (mg)
Totals:								

Blood Glucose Levels			Blood Pressure Levels			Insulin/Medications		
Before:		Time:		(systolic):		Heart Rate (per min)	Type/Units	Pre	Post
After:		Time:		(diastolic):				

Lunch

Meal	Calories	Fat (g)	Carbs (g)	Sugar (g)	Fiber (g)	Net Carb (carbs-fiber)	Protein (g)	Sodium (mg)
Totals:								

Blood Glucose Levels			Blood Pressure Levels			Insulin/Medications		
Before:		Time:		(systolic):		Heart Rate (per min)	Type/Units	Pre	Post
After:		Time:		(diastolic):				

Snack #2

Meal	Calories	Fat (g)	Carbs (g)	Sugar (g)	Fiber (g)	Net Carb (carbs-fiber)	Protein (g)	Sodium (mg)
Totals:								

Blood Glucose Levels			Blood Pressure Levels			Insulin/Medications		
Before:		Time:		(systolic):		Heart Rate (per min)	Type/Units	Pre	Post
After:		Time:		(diastolic):				

Dinner

Meal	Calories	Fat (g)	Carbs (g)	Sugar (g)	Fiber (g)	Net Carb (carbs-fiber)	Protein (g)	Sodium (mg)
Totals:								

Blood Glucose Levels			Blood Pressure Levels			Insulin/Medications		
Before:		Time:		(systolic):		Heart Rate (per min)	Type/Units	Pre	Post
After:		Time:		(diastolic):				

Fasting Blood Sugar:

_____

Water Intake:

total ounces _____

Fitness Log:

Activity	Min

Sleep Log:

Total Hours _____

Notes:

DAILY LOG

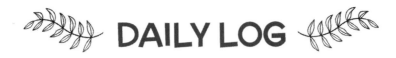

Date: ___/___/_____   **M T W Th F Sa Su**

Breakfast

Meal	Calories	Fat (g)	Carbs (g)	Sugar (g)	Fiber (g)	Net Carb (carbs-fiber)	Protein (g)	Sodium (mg)
Totals:								

Blood Glucose Levels			Blood Pressure Levels			Insulin/Medications		
Before:		Time:	(systolic):	Heart Rate (per min)		Type/Units	Pre	Post
After:		Time:	(diastolic):					

Snack #1

Totals:								

Blood Glucose Levels			Blood Pressure Levels			Insulin/Medications		
Before:		Time:	(systolic):	Heart Rate (per min)		Type/Units	Pre	Post
After:		Time:	(diastolic):					

Lunch

Totals:								

Blood Glucose Levels			Blood Pressure Levels			Insulin/Medications		
Before:		Time:	(systolic):	Heart Rate (per min)		Type/Units	Pre	Post
After:		Time:	(diastolic):					

Snack #2

Totals:								

Blood Glucose Levels			Blood Pressure Levels			Insulin/Medications		
Before:		Time:	(systolic):	Heart Rate (per min)		Type/Units	Pre	Post
After:		Time:	(diastolic):					

Dinner

Totals:								

Blood Glucose Levels			Blood Pressure Levels			Insulin/Medications		
Before:		Time:	(systolic):	Heart Rate (per min)		Type/Units	Pre	Post
After:		Time:	(diastolic):					

Fasting Blood Sugar:

_____

Water Intake:

total ounces _____

Fitness Log:

Activity   Min

Sleep Log:

Total Hours _____

Notes:

DAILY LOG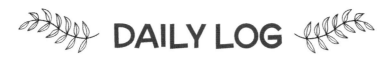

Date: ___/___/_____   M T W Th F Sa Su

Breakfast	Meal		Calories	Fat (g)	Carbs (g)	Sugar (g)	Fiber (g)	Net Carb (carbs-fiber)	Protein (g)	Sodium (mg)
	Totals:									

Blood Glucose Levels			Blood Pressure Levels		Insulin/Medications		
Before:		Time:	(systolic):	Heart Rate (per min)	Type/Units	Pre	Post
After:		Time:	(diastolic):				

Snack #1										
	Totals:									

Blood Glucose Levels			Blood Pressure Levels		Insulin/Medications		
Before:		Time:	(systolic):	Heart Rate (per min)	Type/Units	Pre	Post
After:		Time:	(diastolic):				

Lunch										
	Totals:									

Blood Glucose Levels			Blood Pressure Levels		Insulin/Medications		
Before:		Time:	(systolic):	Heart Rate (per min)	Type/Units	Pre	Post
After:		Time:	(diastolic):				

Snack #2										
	Totals:									

Blood Glucose Levels			Blood Pressure Levels		Insulin/Medications		
Before:		Time:	(systolic):	Heart Rate (per min)	Type/Units	Pre	Post
After:		Time:	(diastolic):				

Dinner										
	Totals:									

Blood Glucose Levels			Blood Pressure Levels		Insulin/Medications		
Before:		Time:	(systolic):	Heart Rate (per min)	Type/Units	Pre	Post
After:		Time:	(diastolic):				

Fasting Blood Sugar:
_____

Water Intake:
total ounces _____

Fitness Log:

Activity	Min

Sleep Log:
Total Hours _____

Notes:
_____
_____
_____
_____
_____
_____
_____
_____
_____
_____

DAILY LOG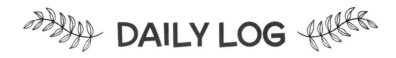

Date: ___/___/_____   **M T W Th F Sa Su**

Breakfast

	Meal	Calories	Fat (g)	Carbs (g)	Sugar (g)	Fiber (g)	Net Carb (carbs-fiber)	Protein (g)	Sodium (mg)
	Totals:								

Blood Glucose Levels				Blood Pressure Levels			Insulin/Medications		
Before:		Time:		(systolic):		Heart Rate (per min)	Type/Units	Pre	Post
After:		Time:		(diastolic):					

Snack #1

	Totals:								

Blood Glucose Levels				Blood Pressure Levels			Insulin/Medications		
Before:		Time:		(systolic):		Heart Rate (per min)	Type/Units	Pre	Post
After:		Time:		(diastolic):					

Lunch

	Totals:								

Blood Glucose Levels				Blood Pressure Levels			Insulin/Medications		
Before:		Time:		(systolic):		Heart Rate (per min)	Type/Units	Pre	Post
After:		Time:		(diastolic):					

Snack #2

	Totals:								

Blood Glucose Levels				Blood Pressure Levels			Insulin/Medications		
Before:		Time:		(systolic):		Heart Rate (per min)	Type/Units	Pre	Post
After:		Time:		(diastolic):					

Dinner

	Totals:								

Blood Glucose Levels				Blood Pressure Levels			Insulin/Medications		
Before:		Time:		(systolic):		Heart Rate (per min)	Type/Units	Pre	Post
After:		Time:		(diastolic):					

Fasting Blood Sugar:

_____

Water Intake:

total ounces _____

Fitness Log:

Activity	Min

Sleep Log:

Total Hours _____

Notes:

_____
_____
_____
_____
_____
_____
_____
_____
_____
_____

DAILY LOG

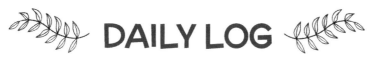

Date: ___/___/_____   **M T W Th F Sa Su**

Breakfast

Meal	Calories	Fat (g)	Carbs (g)	Sugar (g)	Fiber (g)	Net Carb (carbs-fiber)	Protein (g)	Sodium (mg)
Totals:								

Blood Glucose Levels				Blood Pressure Levels			Insulin/Medications		
Before:		Time:		(systolic):		Heart Rate (per min)	Type/Units	Pre	Post
After:		Time:		(diastolic):					

Snack #1

Totals:								

Blood Glucose Levels				Blood Pressure Levels			Insulin/Medications		
Before:		Time:		(systolic):		Heart Rate (per min)	Type/Units	Pre	Post
After:		Time:		(diastolic):					

Lunch

Totals:								

Blood Glucose Levels				Blood Pressure Levels			Insulin/Medications		
Before:		Time:		(systolic):		Heart Rate (per min)	Type/Units	Pre	Post
After:		Time:		(diastolic):					

Snack #2

Totals:								

Blood Glucose Levels				Blood Pressure Levels			Insulin/Medications		
Before:		Time:		(systolic):		Heart Rate (per min)	Type/Units	Pre	Post
After:		Time:		(diastolic):					

Dinner

Totals:								

Blood Glucose Levels				Blood Pressure Levels			Insulin/Medications		
Before:		Time:		(systolic):		Heart Rate (per min)	Type/Units	Pre	Post
After:		Time:		(diastolic):					

Fasting Blood Sugar:
_____

Water Intake:
total ounces _____

Fitness Log:

Activity	Min

Sleep Log:
Total Hours _____

Notes:
_____
_____
_____
_____
_____
_____
_____
_____
_____
_____

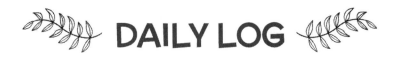

DAILY LOG

Date: ___/___/_____   **M   T   W   Th   F   Sa   Su**

Breakfast

Meal	Calories	Fat (g)	Carbs (g)	Sugar (g)	Fiber (g)	Net Carb (carbs-fiber)	Protein (g)	Sodium (mg)
Totals:								

Blood Glucose Levels			Blood Pressure Levels		Insulin/Medications		
Before:		Time:	(systolic):	Heart Rate (per min)	Type/Units	Pre	Post
After:		Time:	(diastolic):				

Snack #1

Meal	Calories	Fat (g)	Carbs (g)	Sugar (g)	Fiber (g)	Net Carb (carbs-fiber)	Protein (g)	Sodium (mg)
Totals:								

Blood Glucose Levels			Blood Pressure Levels		Insulin/Medications		
Before:		Time:	(systolic):	Heart Rate (per min)	Type/Units	Pre	Post
After:		Time:	(diastolic):				

Lunch

Meal	Calories	Fat (g)	Carbs (g)	Sugar (g)	Fiber (g)	Net Carb (carbs-fiber)	Protein (g)	Sodium (mg)
Totals:								

Blood Glucose Levels			Blood Pressure Levels		Insulin/Medications		
Before:		Time:	(systolic):	Heart Rate (per min)	Type/Units	Pre	Post
After:		Time:	(diastolic):				

Snack #2

Meal	Calories	Fat (g)	Carbs (g)	Sugar (g)	Fiber (g)	Net Carb (carbs-fiber)	Protein (g)	Sodium (mg)
Totals:								

Blood Glucose Levels			Blood Pressure Levels		Insulin/Medications		
Before:		Time:	(systolic):	Heart Rate (per min)	Type/Units	Pre	Post
After:		Time:	(diastolic):				

Dinner

Meal	Calories	Fat (g)	Carbs (g)	Sugar (g)	Fiber (g)	Net Carb (carbs-fiber)	Protein (g)	Sodium (mg)
Totals:								

Blood Glucose Levels			Blood Pressure Levels		Insulin/Medications		
Before:		Time:	(systolic):	Heart Rate (per min)	Type/Units	Pre	Post
After:		Time:	(diastolic):				

Fasting Blood Sugar:

_____

Water Intake:

total ounces _____

Fitness Log:

Activity	Min

Sleep Log:

Total Hours _____

Notes:

DAILY LOG

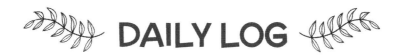

Date: ___/___/_____   **M T W Th F Sa Su**

Breakfast

	Meal	Calories	Fat (g)	Carbs (g)	Sugar (g)	Fiber (g)	Net Carb (carbs-fiber)	Protein (g)	Sodium (mg)
	Totals:								

Blood Glucose Levels			Blood Pressure Levels			Insulin/Medications		
Before:		Time:	(systolic):		Heart Rate (per min)	Type/Units	Pre	Post
After:		Time:	(diastolic):					

Snack #1

	Totals:								

Blood Glucose Levels			Blood Pressure Levels			Insulin/Medications		
Before:		Time:	(systolic):		Heart Rate (per min)	Type/Units	Pre	Post
After:		Time:	(diastolic):					

Lunch

	Totals:								

Blood Glucose Levels			Blood Pressure Levels			Insulin/Medications		
Before:		Time:	(systolic):		Heart Rate (per min)	Type/Units	Pre	Post
After:		Time:	(diastolic):					

Snack #2

	Totals:								

Blood Glucose Levels			Blood Pressure Levels			Insulin/Medications		
Before:		Time:	(systolic):		Heart Rate (per min)	Type/Units	Pre	Post
After:		Time:	(diastolic):					

Dinner

	Totals:								

Blood Glucose Levels			Blood Pressure Levels			Insulin/Medications		
Before:		Time:	(systolic):		Heart Rate (per min)	Type/Units	Pre	Post
After:		Time:	(diastolic):					

Fasting Blood Sugar:

_____

Water Intake:

total ounces _____

Fitness Log:

Activity	Min

Sleep Log:

Total Hours _____

Notes:

_____
_____
_____
_____
_____
_____
_____
_____
_____

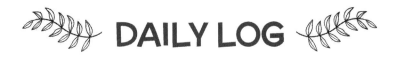

DAILY LOG

Date: ____/____/_____   **M T W Th F Sa Su**

Breakfast

Meal	Calories	Fat (g)	Carbs (g)	Sugar (g)	Fiber (g)	Net Carb (carbs-fiber)	Protein (g)	Sodium (mg)
Totals:								

Blood Glucose Levels				Blood Pressure Levels			Insulin/Medications		
Before:		Time:		(systolic):		Heart Rate (per min)	Type/Units	Pre	Post
After:		Time:		(diastolic):					

Fasting Blood Sugar:

_____

Snack #1

Totals:								

Blood Glucose Levels				Blood Pressure Levels			Insulin/Medications		
Before:		Time:		(systolic):		Heart Rate (per min)	Type/Units	Pre	Post
After:		Time:		(diastolic):					

Water Intake:

total ounces _____

Lunch

Totals:								

Blood Glucose Levels				Blood Pressure Levels			Insulin/Medications		
Before:		Time:		(systolic):		Heart Rate (per min)	Type/Units	Pre	Post
After:		Time:		(diastolic):					

Fitness Log:

Activity	Min

Sleep Log:

Total Hours _____

Snack #2

Totals:								

Blood Glucose Levels				Blood Pressure Levels			Insulin/Medications		
Before:		Time:		(systolic):		Heart Rate (per min)	Type/Units	Pre	Post
After:		Time:		(diastolic):					

Notes:

Dinner

Totals:								

Blood Glucose Levels				Blood Pressure Levels			Insulin/Medications		
Before:		Time:		(systolic):		Heart Rate (per min)	Type/Units	Pre	Post
After:		Time:		(diastolic):					

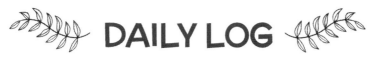

DAILY LOG

Date: ___/___/_____   **M T W Th F Sa Su**

Breakfast

	Meal	Calories	Fat (g)	Carbs (g)	Sugar (g)	Fiber (g)	Net Carb (carbs-fiber)	Protein (g)	Sodium (mg)
	Totals:								

Blood Glucose Levels				Blood Pressure Levels		Heart Rate (per min)	Insulin/Medications		
Before:		Time:		(systolic):			Type/Units	Pre	Post
After:		Time:		(diastolic):					

Snack #1

	Totals:								

Blood Glucose Levels				Blood Pressure Levels		Heart Rate (per min)	Insulin/Medications		
Before:		Time:		(systolic):			Type/Units	Pre	Post
After:		Time:		(diastolic):					

Lunch

	Totals:								

Blood Glucose Levels				Blood Pressure Levels		Heart Rate (per min)	Insulin/Medications		
Before:		Time:		(systolic):			Type/Units	Pre	Post
After:		Time:		(diastolic):					

Snack #2

	Totals:								

Blood Glucose Levels				Blood Pressure Levels		Heart Rate (per min)	Insulin/Medications		
Before:		Time:		(systolic):			Type/Units	Pre	Post
After:		Time:		(diastolic):					

Dinner

	Totals:								

Blood Glucose Levels				Blood Pressure Levels		Heart Rate (per min)	Insulin/Medications		
Before:		Time:		(systolic):			Type/Units	Pre	Post
After:		Time:		(diastolic):					

Fasting Blood Sugar:

_____

Water Intake:

total ounces _____

Fitness Log:

Activity   Min

Sleep Log:

Total Hours _____

Notes:

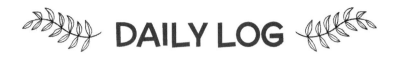

DAILY LOG

Date: ___/___/_____   **M T W Th F Sa Su**

Breakfast

Meal	Calories	Fat (g)	Carbs (g)	Sugar (g)	Fiber (g)	Net Carb (carbs-fiber)	Protein (g)	Sodium (mg)
Totals:								

Blood Glucose Levels				Blood Pressure Levels			Insulin/Medications		
Before:		Time:		(systolic):		Heart Rate (per min)	Type/Units	Pre	Post
After:		Time:		(diastolic):					

Snack #1

Totals:								

Blood Glucose Levels				Blood Pressure Levels			Insulin/Medications		
Before:		Time:		(systolic):		Heart Rate (per min)	Type/Units	Pre	Post
After:		Time:		(diastolic):					

Lunch

Totals:								

Blood Glucose Levels				Blood Pressure Levels			Insulin/Medications		
Before:		Time:		(systolic):		Heart Rate (per min)	Type/Units	Pre	Post
After:		Time:		(diastolic):					

Snack #2

Totals:								

Blood Glucose Levels				Blood Pressure Levels			Insulin/Medications		
Before:		Time:		(systolic):		Heart Rate (per min)	Type/Units	Pre	Post
After:		Time:		(diastolic):					

Dinner

Totals:								

Blood Glucose Levels				Blood Pressure Levels			Insulin/Medications		
Before:		Time:		(systolic):		Heart Rate (per min)	Type/Units	Pre	Post
After:		Time:		(diastolic):					

Fasting Blood Sugar:
_____

Water Intake:
total ounces _____

Fitness Log:

Activity	Min

Sleep Log:
Total Hours _____

Notes:
_____
_____
_____
_____
_____
_____
_____
_____
_____
_____

DAILY LOG

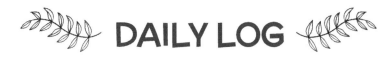

Date: ____/____/_____   **M T W Th F Sa Su**

Breakfast

	Meal	Calories	Fat (g)	Carbs (g)	Sugar (g)	Fiber (g)	Net Carb (carbs-fiber)	Protein (g)	Sodium (mg)
	Totals:								

Blood Glucose Levels			Blood Pressure Levels		Insulin/Medications		
Before:		Time:	(systolic):	Heart Rate (per min)	Type/Units	Pre	Post
After:		Time:	(diastolic):				

Snack #1

	Totals:								

Blood Glucose Levels			Blood Pressure Levels		Insulin/Medications		
Before:		Time:	(systolic):	Heart Rate (per min)	Type/Units	Pre	Post
After:		Time:	(diastolic):				

Lunch

	Totals:								

Blood Glucose Levels			Blood Pressure Levels		Insulin/Medications		
Before:		Time:	(systolic):	Heart Rate (per min)	Type/Units	Pre	Post
After:		Time:	(diastolic):				

Snack #2

	Totals:								

Blood Glucose Levels			Blood Pressure Levels		Insulin/Medications		
Before:		Time:	(systolic):	Heart Rate (per min)	Type/Units	Pre	Post
After:		Time:	(diastolic):				

Dinner

	Totals:								

Blood Glucose Levels			Blood Pressure Levels		Insulin/Medications		
Before:		Time:	(systolic):	Heart Rate (per min)	Type/Units	Pre	Post
After:		Time:	(diastolic):				

Fasting Blood Sugar:
_____

Water Intake:
total ounces _____

Fitness Log:
Activity	Min

Sleep Log:
Total Hours _____

Notes:
_____
_____
_____
_____
_____
_____
_____
_____
_____

DAILY LOG

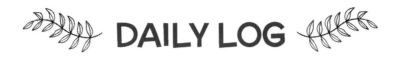

Date: ___/___/_____   **M   T   W   Th   F   Sa   Su**

Breakfast

	Meal	Calories	Fat (g)	Carbs (g)	Sugar (g)	Fiber (g)	Net Carb (carbs-fiber)	Protein (g)	Sodium (mg)
	Totals:								

Blood Glucose Levels				Blood Pressure Levels			Insulin/Medications		
Before:		Time:		(systolic):		Heart Rate (per min)	Type/Units	Pre	Post
After:		Time:		(diastolic):					

Fasting Blood Sugar:

_____

Snack #1

	Totals:								

Blood Glucose Levels				Blood Pressure Levels			Insulin/Medications		
Before:		Time:		(systolic):		Heart Rate (per min)	Type/Units	Pre	Post
After:		Time:		(diastolic):					

Water Intake:

total ounces _____

Lunch

	Totals:								

Blood Glucose Levels				Blood Pressure Levels			Insulin/Medications		
Before:		Time:		(systolic):		Heart Rate (per min)	Type/Units	Pre	Post
After:		Time:		(diastolic):					

Fitness Log:

Activity			Min

Sleep Log:

Total Hours _____

Snack #2

	Totals:								

Blood Glucose Levels				Blood Pressure Levels			Insulin/Medications		
Before:		Time:		(systolic):		Heart Rate (per min)	Type/Units	Pre	Post
After:		Time:		(diastolic):					

Notes:

Dinner

	Totals:								

Blood Glucose Levels				Blood Pressure Levels			Insulin/Medications		
Before:		Time:		(systolic):		Heart Rate (per min)	Type/Units	Pre	Post
After:		Time:		(diastolic):					

DAILY LOG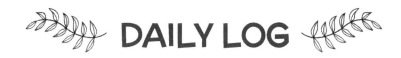

Date: ___/___/_____   **M T W Th F Sa Su**

Breakfast

	Meal	Calories	Fat (g)	Carbs (g)	Sugar (g)	Fiber (g)	Net Carb (carbs-fiber)	Protein (g)	Sodium (mg)
	Totals:								

Blood Glucose Levels			Blood Pressure Levels		Insulin/Medications		
Before:		Time:	(systolic):	Heart Rate (per min)	Type/Units	Pre	Post
After:		Time:	(diastolic):				

Snack #1

	Totals:								

Blood Glucose Levels			Blood Pressure Levels		Insulin/Medications		
Before:		Time:	(systolic):	Heart Rate (per min)	Type/Units	Pre	Post
After:		Time:	(diastolic):				

Lunch

	Totals:								

Blood Glucose Levels			Blood Pressure Levels		Insulin/Medications		
Before:		Time:	(systolic):	Heart Rate (per min)	Type/Units	Pre	Post
After:		Time:	(diastolic):				

Snack #2

	Totals:								

Blood Glucose Levels			Blood Pressure Levels		Insulin/Medications		
Before:		Time:	(systolic):	Heart Rate (per min)	Type/Units	Pre	Post
After:		Time:	(diastolic):				

Dinner

	Totals:								

Blood Glucose Levels			Blood Pressure Levels		Insulin/Medications		
Before:		Time:	(systolic):	Heart Rate (per min)	Type/Units	Pre	Post
After:		Time:	(diastolic):				

Fasting Blood Sugar:

_____

Water Intake:

total ounces _____

Fitness Log:

Activity	Min

Sleep Log:

Total Hours _____

Notes:

DAILY LOG

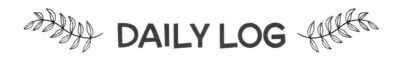

Date: ___/___/_____   **M T W Th F Sa Su**

Breakfast

Meal	Calories	Fat (g)	Carbs (g)	Sugar (g)	Fiber (g)	Net Carb (carbs-fiber)	Protein (g)	Sodium (mg)
Totals:								

Blood Glucose Levels			Blood Pressure Levels			Insulin/Medications		
Before:		Time:	(systolic):		Heart Rate (per min)	Type/Units	Pre	Post
After:		Time:	(diastolic):					

Snack #1

Totals:								

Blood Glucose Levels			Blood Pressure Levels			Insulin/Medications		
Before:		Time:	(systolic):		Heart Rate (per min)	Type/Units	Pre	Post
After:		Time:	(diastolic):					

Lunch

Totals:								

Blood Glucose Levels			Blood Pressure Levels			Insulin/Medications		
Before:		Time:	(systolic):		Heart Rate (per min)	Type/Units	Pre	Post
After:		Time:	(diastolic):					

Snack #2

Totals:								

Blood Glucose Levels			Blood Pressure Levels			Insulin/Medications		
Before:		Time:	(systolic):		Heart Rate (per min)	Type/Units	Pre	Post
After:		Time:	(diastolic):					

Dinner

Totals:								

Blood Glucose Levels			Blood Pressure Levels			Insulin/Medications		
Before:		Time:	(systolic):		Heart Rate (per min)	Type/Units	Pre	Post
After:		Time:	(diastolic):					

Fasting Blood Sugar:

_____

Water Intake:

🍶 🍶 🍶 🍶 🍶 🍶 🍶 🍶

total ounces _____

Fitness Log:

Activity	Min

Sleep Log:

Total Hours _____

Notes:

_____
_____
_____
_____
_____
_____
_____
_____
_____
_____
_____

DAILY LOG
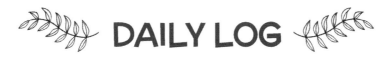

Date: ____/____/_____

M T W Th F Sa Su

Breakfast

	Meal	Calories	Fat (g)	Carbs (g)	Sugar (g)	Fiber (g)	Net Carb (carbs-fiber)	Protein (g)	Sodium (mg)
	Totals:								

Blood Glucose Levels				Blood Pressure Levels			Insulin/Medications		
Before:		Time:		(systolic):		Heart Rate (per min)	Type/Units	Pre	Post
After:		Time:		(diastolic):					

Snack #1

	Totals:								

Blood Glucose Levels				Blood Pressure Levels			Insulin/Medications		
Before:		Time:		(systolic):		Heart Rate (per min)	Type/Units	Pre	Post
After:		Time:		(diastolic):					

Lunch

	Totals:								

Blood Glucose Levels				Blood Pressure Levels			Insulin/Medications		
Before:		Time:		(systolic):		Heart Rate (per min)	Type/Units	Pre	Post
After:		Time:		(diastolic):					

Snack #2

	Totals:								

Blood Glucose Levels				Blood Pressure Levels			Insulin/Medications		
Before:		Time:		(systolic):		Heart Rate (per min)	Type/Units	Pre	Post
After:		Time:		(diastolic):					

Dinner

	Totals:								

Blood Glucose Levels				Blood Pressure Levels			Insulin/Medications		
Before:		Time:		(systolic):		Heart Rate (per min)	Type/Units	Pre	Post
After:		Time:		(diastolic):					

Fasting Blood Sugar:

_____

Water Intake:

total ounces _____

Fitness Log:

Activity	Min

Sleep Log:

Total Hours _____

Notes:

_____
_____
_____
_____
_____
_____
_____
_____
_____

DAILY LOG

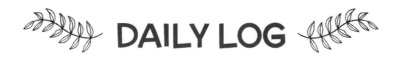

Date: ___/___/_____   **M T W Th F Sa Su**

Breakfast

	Meal	Calories	Fat (g)	Carbs (g)	Sugar (g)	Fiber (g)	Net Carb (carbs-fiber)	Protein (g)	Sodium (mg)
	Totals:								

Blood Glucose Levels				Blood Pressure Levels			Insulin/Medications		
Before:		Time:		(systolic):		Heart Rate (per min)	Type/Units	Pre	Post
After:		Time:		(diastolic):					

Fasting Blood Sugar:

_____

Snack #1

	Totals:								

Blood Glucose Levels				Blood Pressure Levels			Insulin/Medications		
Before:		Time:		(systolic):		Heart Rate (per min)	Type/Units	Pre	Post
After:		Time:		(diastolic):					

Water Intake:

🍶🍶🍶🍶🍶🍶🍶🍶🍶

total ounces _____

Lunch

	Totals:								

Blood Glucose Levels				Blood Pressure Levels			Insulin/Medications		
Before:		Time:		(systolic):		Heart Rate (per min)	Type/Units	Pre	Post
After:		Time:		(diastolic):					

Fitness Log:

Activity   Min

Sleep Log:

Total Hours _____

Snack #2

	Totals:								

Blood Glucose Levels				Blood Pressure Levels			Insulin/Medications		
Before:		Time:		(systolic):		Heart Rate (per min)	Type/Units	Pre	Post
After:		Time:		(diastolic):					

Notes:

Dinner

	Totals:								

Blood Glucose Levels				Blood Pressure Levels			Insulin/Medications		
Before:		Time:		(systolic):		Heart Rate (per min)	Type/Units	Pre	Post
After:		Time:		(diastolic):					

DAILY LOG

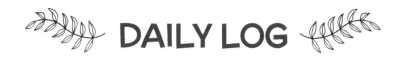

Date: _____/_____/_____   M T W Th F Sa Su

Breakfast

Meal	Calories	Fat (g)	Carbs (g)	Sugar (g)	Fiber (g)	Net Carb (carbs-fiber)	Protein (g)	Sodium (mg)
Totals:								

Blood Glucose Levels				Blood Pressure Levels			Insulin/Medications		
Before:		Time:		(systolic):		Heart Rate (per min)	Type/Units	Pre	Post
After:		Time:		(diastolic):					

Snack #1

Meal	Calories	Fat (g)	Carbs (g)	Sugar (g)	Fiber (g)	Net Carb (carbs-fiber)	Protein (g)	Sodium (mg)
Totals:								

Blood Glucose Levels				Blood Pressure Levels			Insulin/Medications		
Before:		Time:		(systolic):		Heart Rate (per min)	Type/Units	Pre	Post
After:		Time:		(diastolic):					

Lunch

Meal	Calories	Fat (g)	Carbs (g)	Sugar (g)	Fiber (g)	Net Carb (carbs-fiber)	Protein (g)	Sodium (mg)
Totals:								

Blood Glucose Levels				Blood Pressure Levels			Insulin/Medications		
Before:		Time:		(systolic):		Heart Rate (per min)	Type/Units	Pre	Post
After:		Time:		(diastolic):					

Snack #2

Meal	Calories	Fat (g)	Carbs (g)	Sugar (g)	Fiber (g)	Net Carb (carbs-fiber)	Protein (g)	Sodium (mg)
Totals:								

Blood Glucose Levels				Blood Pressure Levels			Insulin/Medications		
Before:		Time:		(systolic):		Heart Rate (per min)	Type/Units	Pre	Post
After:		Time:		(diastolic):					

Dinner

Meal	Calories	Fat (g)	Carbs (g)	Sugar (g)	Fiber (g)	Net Carb (carbs-fiber)	Protein (g)	Sodium (mg)
Totals:								

Blood Glucose Levels				Blood Pressure Levels			Insulin/Medications		
Before:		Time:		(systolic):		Heart Rate (per min)	Type/Units	Pre	Post
After:		Time:		(diastolic):					

Fasting Blood Sugar:

_____

Water Intake:

total ounces _____

Fitness Log:

Activity	Min

Sleep Log:

Total Hours _____

Notes:

_____
_____
_____
_____
_____
_____
_____
_____
_____
_____
_____
_____

DAILY LOG
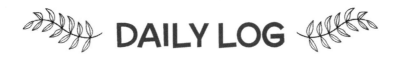

Date: ___/___/_____   **M   T   W   Th   F   Sa   Su**

Breakfast

	Meal	Calories	Fat (g)	Carbs (g)	Sugar (g)	Fiber (g)	Net Carb (carbs-fiber)	Protein (g)	Sodium (mg)
	Totals:								

Blood Glucose Levels			Blood Pressure Levels		Insulin/Medications		
Before:		Time:	(systolic):	Heart Rate (per min)	Type/Units	Pre	Post
After:		Time:	(diastolic):				

Fasting Blood Sugar:

_____

Snack #1

	Totals:								

Blood Glucose Levels			Blood Pressure Levels		Insulin/Medications		
Before:		Time:	(systolic):	Heart Rate (per min)	Type/Units	Pre	Post
After:		Time:	(diastolic):				

Water Intake:

total ounces _____

Lunch

	Totals:								

Blood Glucose Levels			Blood Pressure Levels		Insulin/Medications		
Before:		Time:	(systolic):	Heart Rate (per min)	Type/Units	Pre	Post
After:		Time:	(diastolic):				

Fitness Log:

Activity	Min

Sleep Log:

Total Hours _____

Snack #2

	Totals:								

Blood Glucose Levels			Blood Pressure Levels		Insulin/Medications		
Before:		Time:	(systolic):	Heart Rate (per min)	Type/Units	Pre	Post
After:		Time:	(diastolic):				

Notes:

Dinner

	Totals:								

Blood Glucose Levels			Blood Pressure Levels		Insulin/Medications		
Before:		Time:	(systolic):	Heart Rate (per min)	Type/Units	Pre	Post
After:		Time:	(diastolic):				

DAILY LOG

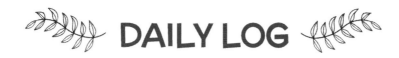

Date: ___/___/_____   **M T W Th F Sa Su**

Breakfast

	Meal	Calories	Fat (g)	Carbs (g)	Sugar (g)	Fiber (g)	Net Carb (carbs-fiber)	Protein (g)	Sodium (mg)
	Totals:								

Blood Glucose Levels			Blood Pressure Levels			Insulin/Medications		
Before:		Time:	(systolic):		Heart Rate (per min)	Type/Units	Pre	Post
After:		Time:	(diastolic):					

Snack #1

	Totals:								

Blood Glucose Levels			Blood Pressure Levels			Insulin/Medications		
Before:		Time:	(systolic):		Heart Rate (per min)	Type/Units	Pre	Post
After:		Time:	(diastolic):					

Lunch

	Totals:								

Blood Glucose Levels			Blood Pressure Levels			Insulin/Medications		
Before:		Time:	(systolic):		Heart Rate (per min)	Type/Units	Pre	Post
After:		Time:	(diastolic):					

Snack #2

	Totals:								

Blood Glucose Levels			Blood Pressure Levels			Insulin/Medications		
Before:		Time:	(systolic):		Heart Rate (per min)	Type/Units	Pre	Post
After:		Time:	(diastolic):					

Dinner

	Totals:								

Blood Glucose Levels			Blood Pressure Levels			Insulin/Medications		
Before:		Time:	(systolic):		Heart Rate (per min)	Type/Units	Pre	Post
After:		Time:	(diastolic):					

Fasting Blood Sugar:

_____

Water Intake:

🍼 🍼 🍼 🍼 🍼 🍼 🍼 🍼

total ounces _____

Fitness Log:

Activity	Min

Sleep Log:

Total Hours _____

Notes:

_____
_____
_____
_____
_____
_____
_____
_____

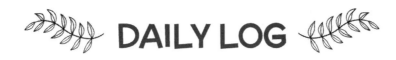

DAILY LOG

Date: ___/___/_____   **M T W Th F Sa Su**

Breakfast

Meal	Calories	Fat (g)	Carbs (g)	Sugar (g)	Fiber (g)	Net Carb (carbs-fiber)	Protein (g)	Sodium (mg)
Totals:								

Blood Glucose Levels		Blood Pressure Levels		Insulin/Medications		
Before:	Time:	(systolic):	Heart Rate (per min)	Type/Units	Pre	Post
After:	Time:	(diastolic):				

Snack #1

Totals:								

Blood Glucose Levels		Blood Pressure Levels		Insulin/Medications		
Before:	Time:	(systolic):	Heart Rate (per min)	Type/Units	Pre	Post
After:	Time:	(diastolic):				

Lunch

Totals:								

Blood Glucose Levels		Blood Pressure Levels		Insulin/Medications		
Before:	Time:	(systolic):	Heart Rate (per min)	Type/Units	Pre	Post
After:	Time:	(diastolic):				

Snack #2

Totals:								

Blood Glucose Levels		Blood Pressure Levels		Insulin/Medications		
Before:	Time:	(systolic):	Heart Rate (per min)	Type/Units	Pre	Post
After:	Time:	(diastolic):				

Dinner

Totals:								

Blood Glucose Levels		Blood Pressure Levels		Insulin/Medications		
Before:	Time:	(systolic):	Heart Rate (per min)	Type/Units	Pre	Post
After:	Time:	(diastolic):				

Fasting Blood Sugar:
_____

Water Intake:
total ounces _____

Fitness Log:
Activity	Min

Sleep Log:
Total Hours _____

Notes:

DAILY LOG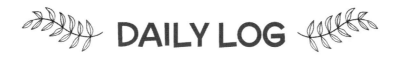

Date: ___/___/_____   **M   T   W   Th   F   Sa   Su**

Breakfast

Meal	Calories	Fat (g)	Carbs (g)	Sugar (g)	Fiber (g)	Net Carb (carbs-fiber)	Protein (g)	Sodium (mg)
Totals:								

Blood Glucose Levels			Blood Pressure Levels		Insulin/Medications		
Before:		Time:	(systolic):	Heart Rate (per min)	Type/Units	Pre	Post
After:		Time:	(diastolic):				

Fasting Blood Sugar:
_____

Snack #1

Totals:								

Blood Glucose Levels			Blood Pressure Levels		Insulin/Medications		
Before:		Time:	(systolic):	Heart Rate (per min)	Type/Units	Pre	Post
After:		Time:	(diastolic):				

Water Intake:
total ounces _____

Fitness Log:

Activity	Min

Lunch

Totals:								

Blood Glucose Levels			Blood Pressure Levels		Insulin/Medications		
Before:		Time:	(systolic):	Heart Rate (per min)	Type/Units	Pre	Post
After:		Time:	(diastolic):				

Sleep Log:
Total Hours _____

Snack #2

Totals:								

Blood Glucose Levels			Blood Pressure Levels		Insulin/Medications		
Before:		Time:	(systolic):	Heart Rate (per min)	Type/Units	Pre	Post
After:		Time:	(diastolic):				

Notes:

Dinner

Totals:								

Blood Glucose Levels			Blood Pressure Levels		Insulin/Medications		
Before:		Time:	(systolic):	Heart Rate (per min)	Type/Units	Pre	Post
After:		Time:	(diastolic):				

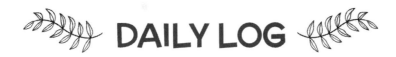

DAILY LOG

Date: ___/___/_____   **M T W Th F Sa Su**

Breakfast

Meal	Calories	Fat (g)	Carbs (g)	Sugar (g)	Fiber (g)	Net Carb (carbs-fiber)	Protein (g)	Sodium (mg)
Totals:								

Blood Glucose Levels				Blood Pressure Levels			Insulin/Medications		
Before:		Time:		(systolic):		Heart Rate (per min)	Type/Units	Pre	Post
After:		Time:		(diastolic):					

Snack #1

Totals:								

Blood Glucose Levels				Blood Pressure Levels			Insulin/Medications		
Before:		Time:		(systolic):		Heart Rate (per min)	Type/Units	Pre	Post
After:		Time:		(diastolic):					

Lunch

Totals:								

Blood Glucose Levels				Blood Pressure Levels			Insulin/Medications		
Before:		Time:		(systolic):		Heart Rate (per min)	Type/Units	Pre	Post
After:		Time:		(diastolic):					

Snack #2

Totals:								

Blood Glucose Levels				Blood Pressure Levels			Insulin/Medications		
Before:		Time:		(systolic):		Heart Rate (per min)	Type/Units	Pre	Post
After:		Time:		(diastolic):					

Dinner

Totals:								

Blood Glucose Levels				Blood Pressure Levels			Insulin/Medications		
Before:		Time:		(systolic):		Heart Rate (per min)	Type/Units	Pre	Post
After:		Time:		(diastolic):					

Fasting Blood Sugar:

_____

Water Intake:

total ounces _____

Fitness Log:

Activity	Min

Sleep Log:

Total Hours _____

Notes:

_____
_____
_____
_____
_____
_____
_____
_____
_____

DAILY LOG

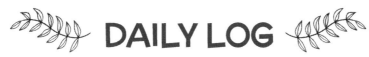

Date: ___/___/_____   **M T W Th F Sa Su**

Breakfast

	Meal	Calories	Fat (g)	Carbs (g)	Sugar (g)	Fiber (g)	Net Carb (carbs-fiber)	Protein (g)	Sodium (mg)
	Totals:								

Blood Glucose Levels				Blood Pressure Levels			Insulin/Medications		
Before:		Time:		(systolic):		Heart Rate (per min)	Type/Units	Pre	Post
After:		Time:		(diastolic):					

Snack #1

	Totals:								

Blood Glucose Levels				Blood Pressure Levels			Insulin/Medications		
Before:		Time:		(systolic):		Heart Rate (per min)	Type/Units	Pre	Post
After:		Time:		(diastolic):					

Lunch

	Totals:								

Blood Glucose Levels				Blood Pressure Levels			Insulin/Medications		
Before:		Time:		(systolic):		Heart Rate (per min)	Type/Units	Pre	Post
After:		Time:		(diastolic):					

Snack #2

	Totals:								

Blood Glucose Levels				Blood Pressure Levels			Insulin/Medications		
Before:		Time:		(systolic):		Heart Rate (per min)	Type/Units	Pre	Post
After:		Time:		(diastolic):					

Dinner

	Totals:								

Blood Glucose Levels				Blood Pressure Levels			Insulin/Medications		
Before:		Time:		(systolic):		Heart Rate (per min)	Type/Units	Pre	Post
After:		Time:		(diastolic):					

Fasting Blood Sugar:
_____

Water Intake:
total ounces _____

Fitness Log:
Activity	Min

Sleep Log:
Total Hours _____

Notes:
_____
_____
_____
_____
_____
_____
_____
_____
_____

DAILY LOG

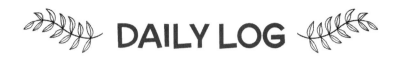

Date: ___/___/_____   **M T W Th F Sa Su**

Breakfast

Meal	Calories	Fat (g)	Carbs (g)	Sugar (g)	Fiber (g)	Net Carb (carbs-fiber)	Protein (g)	Sodium (mg)
Totals:								

Blood Glucose Levels			Blood Pressure Levels			Insulin/Medications		
Before:		Time:	(systolic):		Heart Rate (per min)	Type/Units	Pre	Post
After:		Time:	(diastolic):					

Snack #1

Meal	Calories	Fat (g)	Carbs (g)	Sugar (g)	Fiber (g)	Net Carb (carbs-fiber)	Protein (g)	Sodium (mg)
Totals:								

Blood Glucose Levels			Blood Pressure Levels			Insulin/Medications		
Before:		Time:	(systolic):		Heart Rate (per min)	Type/Units	Pre	Post
After:		Time:	(diastolic):					

Lunch

Meal	Calories	Fat (g)	Carbs (g)	Sugar (g)	Fiber (g)	Net Carb (carbs-fiber)	Protein (g)	Sodium (mg)
Totals:								

Blood Glucose Levels			Blood Pressure Levels			Insulin/Medications		
Before:		Time:	(systolic):		Heart Rate (per min)	Type/Units	Pre	Post
After:		Time:	(diastolic):					

Snack #2

Meal	Calories	Fat (g)	Carbs (g)	Sugar (g)	Fiber (g)	Net Carb (carbs-fiber)	Protein (g)	Sodium (mg)
Totals:								

Blood Glucose Levels			Blood Pressure Levels			Insulin/Medications		
Before:		Time:	(systolic):		Heart Rate (per min)	Type/Units	Pre	Post
After:		Time:	(diastolic):					

Dinner

Meal	Calories	Fat (g)	Carbs (g)	Sugar (g)	Fiber (g)	Net Carb (carbs-fiber)	Protein (g)	Sodium (mg)
Totals:								

Blood Glucose Levels			Blood Pressure Levels			Insulin/Medications		
Before:		Time:	(systolic):		Heart Rate (per min)	Type/Units	Pre	Post
After:		Time:	(diastolic):					

Fasting Blood Sugar:

_____

Water Intake:

total ounces _____

Fitness Log:

Activity	Min

Sleep Log:

Total Hours _____

Notes:

DAILY LOG

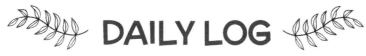

Date: ___/___/_____   **M T W Th F Sa Su**

Breakfast

	Meal	Calories	Fat (g)	Carbs (g)	Sugar (g)	Fiber (g)	Net Carb (carbs-fiber)	Protein (g)	Sodium (mg)
	Totals:								

Blood Glucose Levels				Blood Pressure Levels			Insulin/Medications		
Before:		Time:		(systolic):		Heart Rate (per min)	Type/Units	Pre	Post
After:		Time:		(diastolic):					

Snack #1

	Totals:								

Blood Glucose Levels				Blood Pressure Levels			Insulin/Medications		
Before:		Time:		(systolic):		Heart Rate (per min)	Type/Units	Pre	Post
After:		Time:		(diastolic):					

Lunch

	Totals:								

Blood Glucose Levels				Blood Pressure Levels			Insulin/Medications		
Before:		Time:		(systolic):		Heart Rate (per min)	Type/Units	Pre	Post
After:		Time:		(diastolic):					

Snack #2

	Totals:								

Blood Glucose Levels				Blood Pressure Levels			Insulin/Medications		
Before:		Time:		(systolic):		Heart Rate (per min)	Type/Units	Pre	Post
After:		Time:		(diastolic):					

Dinner

	Totals:								

Blood Glucose Levels				Blood Pressure Levels			Insulin/Medications		
Before:		Time:		(systolic):		Heart Rate (per min)	Type/Units	Pre	Post
After:		Time:		(diastolic):					

Fasting Blood Sugar:

_____

Water Intake:

🍶🍶🍶🍶🍶🍶🍶🍶

total ounces _____

Fitness Log:

Activity	Min

Sleep Log:

Total Hours _____

Notes:

_____
_____
_____
_____
_____
_____
_____
_____
_____

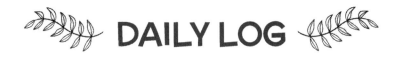

DAILY LOG

Date: ___/___/_____   M T W Th F Sa Su

Breakfast

Meal	Calories	Fat (g)	Carbs (g)	Sugar (g)	Fiber (g)	Net Carb (carbs-fiber)	Protein (g)	Sodium (mg)
Totals:								

Blood Glucose Levels			Blood Pressure Levels			Insulin/Medications		
Before:		Time:	(systolic):		Heart Rate (per min)	Type/Units	Pre	Post
After:		Time:	(diastolic):					

Snack #1

Meal	Calories	Fat (g)	Carbs (g)	Sugar (g)	Fiber (g)	Net Carb (carbs-fiber)	Protein (g)	Sodium (mg)
Totals:								

Blood Glucose Levels			Blood Pressure Levels			Insulin/Medications		
Before:		Time:	(systolic):		Heart Rate (per min)	Type/Units	Pre	Post
After:		Time:	(diastolic):					

Lunch

Meal	Calories	Fat (g)	Carbs (g)	Sugar (g)	Fiber (g)	Net Carb (carbs-fiber)	Protein (g)	Sodium (mg)
Totals:								

Blood Glucose Levels			Blood Pressure Levels			Insulin/Medications		
Before:		Time:	(systolic):		Heart Rate (per min)	Type/Units	Pre	Post
After:		Time:	(diastolic):					

Snack #2

Meal	Calories	Fat (g)	Carbs (g)	Sugar (g)	Fiber (g)	Net Carb (carbs-fiber)	Protein (g)	Sodium (mg)
Totals:								

Blood Glucose Levels			Blood Pressure Levels			Insulin/Medications		
Before:		Time:	(systolic):		Heart Rate (per min)	Type/Units	Pre	Post
After:		Time:	(diastolic):					

Dinner

Meal	Calories	Fat (g)	Carbs (g)	Sugar (g)	Fiber (g)	Net Carb (carbs-fiber)	Protein (g)	Sodium (mg)
Totals:								

Blood Glucose Levels			Blood Pressure Levels			Insulin/Medications		
Before:		Time:	(systolic):		Heart Rate (per min)	Type/Units	Pre	Post
After:		Time:	(diastolic):					

Fasting Blood Sugar:

_____

Water Intake:

total ounces _____

Fitness Log:

Activity	Min

Sleep Log:

Total Hours _____

Notes:

DAILY LOG

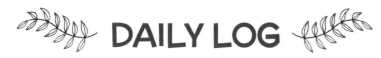

Date: ____/____/_____   **M T W Th F Sa Su**

Breakfast

	Meal	Calories	Fat (g)	Carbs (g)	Sugar (g)	Fiber (g)	Net Carb (carbs-fiber)	Protein (g)	Sodium (mg)
	Totals:								

Blood Glucose Levels				Blood Pressure Levels			Insulin/Medications		
Before:		Time:		(systolic):		Heart Rate (per min)	Type/Units	Pre	Post
After:		Time:		(diastolic):					

Snack #1

	Totals:								

Blood Glucose Levels				Blood Pressure Levels			Insulin/Medications		
Before:		Time:		(systolic):		Heart Rate (per min)	Type/Units	Pre	Post
After:		Time:		(diastolic):					

Lunch

	Totals:								

Blood Glucose Levels				Blood Pressure Levels			Insulin/Medications		
Before:		Time:		(systolic):		Heart Rate (per min)	Type/Units	Pre	Post
After:		Time:		(diastolic):					

Snack #2

	Totals:								

Blood Glucose Levels				Blood Pressure Levels			Insulin/Medications		
Before:		Time:		(systolic):		Heart Rate (per min)	Type/Units	Pre	Post
After:		Time:		(diastolic):					

Dinner

	Totals:								

Blood Glucose Levels				Blood Pressure Levels			Insulin/Medications		
Before:		Time:		(systolic):		Heart Rate (per min)	Type/Units	Pre	Post
After:		Time:		(diastolic):					

Fasting Blood Sugar:

_____

Water Intake:

total ounces _____

Fitness Log:

Activity	Min

Sleep Log:

Total Hours _____

Notes:

DAILY LOG

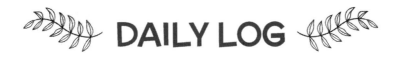

Date: ___/___/_____   **M T W Th F Sa Su**

Breakfast

Meal	Calories	Fat (g)	Carbs (g)	Sugar (g)	Fiber (g)	Net Carb (carbs-fiber)	Protein (g)	Sodium (mg)
Totals:								

Blood Glucose Levels				Blood Pressure Levels			Insulin/Medications		
Before:		Time:		(systolic):		Heart Rate (per min)	Type/Units	Pre	Post
After:		Time:		(diastolic):					

Snack #1

Meal	Calories	Fat (g)	Carbs (g)	Sugar (g)	Fiber (g)	Net Carb (carbs-fiber)	Protein (g)	Sodium (mg)
Totals:								

Blood Glucose Levels				Blood Pressure Levels			Insulin/Medications		
Before:		Time:		(systolic):		Heart Rate (per min)	Type/Units	Pre	Post
After:		Time:		(diastolic):					

Lunch

Meal	Calories	Fat (g)	Carbs (g)	Sugar (g)	Fiber (g)	Net Carb (carbs-fiber)	Protein (g)	Sodium (mg)
Totals:								

Blood Glucose Levels				Blood Pressure Levels			Insulin/Medications		
Before:		Time:		(systolic):		Heart Rate (per min)	Type/Units	Pre	Post
After:		Time:		(diastolic):					

Snack #2

Meal	Calories	Fat (g)	Carbs (g)	Sugar (g)	Fiber (g)	Net Carb (carbs-fiber)	Protein (g)	Sodium (mg)
Totals:								

Blood Glucose Levels				Blood Pressure Levels			Insulin/Medications		
Before:		Time:		(systolic):		Heart Rate (per min)	Type/Units	Pre	Post
After:		Time:		(diastolic):					

Dinner

Meal	Calories	Fat (g)	Carbs (g)	Sugar (g)	Fiber (g)	Net Carb (carbs-fiber)	Protein (g)	Sodium (mg)
Totals:								

Blood Glucose Levels				Blood Pressure Levels			Insulin/Medications		
Before:		Time:		(systolic):		Heart Rate (per min)	Type/Units	Pre	Post
After:		Time:		(diastolic):					

Fasting Blood Sugar:

_____

Water Intake:

total ounces _____

Fitness Log:

Activity	Min

Sleep Log:

Total Hours _____

Notes:

DAILY LOG

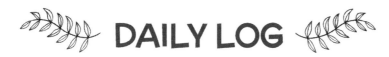

Date: ___/___/_____   **M T W Th F Sa Su**

Breakfast

Meal	Calories	Fat (g)	Carbs (g)	Sugar (g)	Fiber (g)	Net Carb (carbs-fiber)	Protein (g)	Sodium (mg)
Totals:								

Blood Glucose Levels		Blood Pressure Levels		Insulin/Medications		
Before:	Time:	(systolic):	Heart Rate (per min)	Type/Units	Pre	Post
After:	Time:	(diastolic):				

Snack #1

Totals:								

Blood Glucose Levels		Blood Pressure Levels		Insulin/Medications		
Before:	Time:	(systolic):	Heart Rate (per min)	Type/Units	Pre	Post
After:	Time:	(diastolic):				

Lunch

Totals:								

Blood Glucose Levels		Blood Pressure Levels		Insulin/Medications		
Before:	Time:	(systolic):	Heart Rate (per min)	Type/Units	Pre	Post
After:	Time:	(diastolic):				

Snack #2

Totals:								

Blood Glucose Levels		Blood Pressure Levels		Insulin/Medications		
Before:	Time:	(systolic):	Heart Rate (per min)	Type/Units	Pre	Post
After:	Time:	(diastolic):				

Dinner

Totals:								

Blood Glucose Levels		Blood Pressure Levels		Insulin/Medications		
Before:	Time:	(systolic):	Heart Rate (per min)	Type/Units	Pre	Post
After:	Time:	(diastolic):				

Fasting Blood Sugar:

_____

Water Intake:

total ounces _____

Fitness Log:

Activity	Min

Sleep Log:

Total Hours _____

Notes:

_____
_____
_____
_____
_____
_____
_____
_____
_____
_____

DAILY LOG

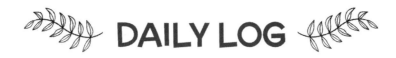

Date: ___/___/_____   **M T W Th F Sa Su**

Breakfast

Meal	Calories	Fat (g)	Carbs (g)	Sugar (g)	Fiber (g)	Net Carb (carbs-fiber)	Protein (g)	Sodium (mg)
Totals:								

Blood Glucose Levels			Blood Pressure Levels			Insulin/Medications		
Before:		Time:	(systolic):		Heart Rate (per min)	Type/Units	Pre	Post
After:		Time:	(diastolic):					

Snack #1

Totals:								

Blood Glucose Levels			Blood Pressure Levels			Insulin/Medications		
Before:		Time:	(systolic):		Heart Rate (per min)	Type/Units	Pre	Post
After:		Time:	(diastolic):					

Lunch

Totals:								

Blood Glucose Levels			Blood Pressure Levels			Insulin/Medications		
Before:		Time:	(systolic):		Heart Rate (per min)	Type/Units	Pre	Post
After:		Time:	(diastolic):					

Snack #2

Totals:								

Blood Glucose Levels			Blood Pressure Levels			Insulin/Medications		
Before:		Time:	(systolic):		Heart Rate (per min)	Type/Units	Pre	Post
After:		Time:	(diastolic):					

Dinner

Totals:								

Blood Glucose Levels			Blood Pressure Levels			Insulin/Medications		
Before:		Time:	(systolic):		Heart Rate (per min)	Type/Units	Pre	Post
After:		Time:	(diastolic):					

Fasting Blood Sugar:

_____

Water Intake:

total ounces _____

Fitness Log:

Activity	Min

Sleep Log:

Total Hours _____

Notes:

_____
_____
_____
_____
_____
_____
_____
_____
_____
_____

DAILY LOG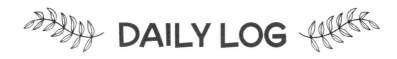

Date: ___/___/_____ **M T W Th F Sa Su**

Breakfast

	Meal	Calories	Fat (g)	Carbs (g)	Sugar (g)	Fiber (g)	Net Carb (carbs-fiber)	Protein (g)	Sodium (mg)
	Totals:								

Blood Glucose Levels				Blood Pressure Levels			Insulin/Medications		
Before:		Time:		(systolic):		Heart Rate (per min)	Type/Units	Pre	Post
After:		Time:		(diastolic):					

Snack #1

	Totals:								

Blood Glucose Levels				Blood Pressure Levels			Insulin/Medications		
Before:		Time:		(systolic):		Heart Rate (per min)	Type/Units	Pre	Post
After:		Time:		(diastolic):					

Lunch

	Totals:								

Blood Glucose Levels				Blood Pressure Levels			Insulin/Medications		
Before:		Time:		(systolic):		Heart Rate (per min)	Type/Units	Pre	Post
After:		Time:		(diastolic):					

Snack #2

	Totals:								

Blood Glucose Levels				Blood Pressure Levels			Insulin/Medications		
Before:		Time:		(systolic):		Heart Rate (per min)	Type/Units	Pre	Post
After:		Time:		(diastolic):					

Dinner

	Totals:								

Blood Glucose Levels				Blood Pressure Levels			Insulin/Medications		
Before:		Time:		(systolic):		Heart Rate (per min)	Type/Units	Pre	Post
After:		Time:		(diastolic):					

Fasting Blood Sugar:
_____

Water Intake:
total ounces _____

Fitness Log:

Activity	Min

Sleep Log:
Total Hours _____

Notes:

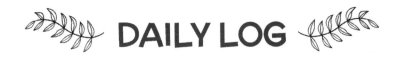

DAILY LOG

Date: ___/___/_____   **M T W Th F Sa Su**

Breakfast

Meal	Calories	Fat (g)	Carbs (g)	Sugar (g)	Fiber (g)	Net Carb (carbs-fiber)	Protein (g)	Sodium (mg)
Totals:								

Blood Glucose Levels

Before:		Time:	
After:		Time:	

Blood Pressure Levels

(systolic):		Heart Rate (per min)	
(diastolic):			

Insulin/Medications

Type/Units	Pre	Post

Snack #1

Totals:								

Blood Glucose Levels

Before:		Time:	
After:		Time:	

Blood Pressure Levels

(systolic):		Heart Rate (per min)	
(diastolic):			

Insulin/Medications

Type/Units	Pre	Post

Lunch

Totals:								

Blood Glucose Levels

Before:		Time:	
After:		Time:	

Blood Pressure Levels

(systolic):		Heart Rate (per min)	
(diastolic):			

Insulin/Medications

Type/Units	Pre	Post

Snack #2

Totals:								

Blood Glucose Levels

Before:		Time:	
After:		Time:	

Blood Pressure Levels

(systolic):		Heart Rate (per min)	
(diastolic):			

Insulin/Medications

Type/Units	Pre	Post

Dinner

Totals:								

Blood Glucose Levels

Before:		Time:	
After:		Time:	

Blood Pressure Levels

(systolic):		Heart Rate (per min)	
(diastolic):			

Insulin/Medications

Type/Units	Pre	Post

Fasting Blood Sugar:

_____

Water Intake:

total ounces _____

Fitness Log:

Activity	Min

Sleep Log:

Total Hours _____

Notes:

DAILY LOG

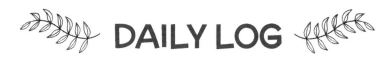

Date: ___/___/_____   **M T W Th F Sa Su**

Breakfast

Meal	Calories	Fat (g)	Carbs (g)	Sugar (g)	Fiber (g)	Net Carb (carbs-fiber)	Protein (g)	Sodium (mg)
Totals:								

Blood Glucose Levels		Blood Pressure Levels		Insulin/Medications		
				Heart Rate (per min)	Type/Units	Pre	Post
Before:	Time:	(systolic):					
After:	Time:	(diastolic):					

Snack #1

Totals:								

Blood Glucose Levels		Blood Pressure Levels		Insulin/Medications		
				Heart Rate (per min)	Type/Units	Pre	Post
Before:	Time:	(systolic):					
After:	Time:	(diastolic):					

Lunch

Totals:								

Blood Glucose Levels		Blood Pressure Levels		Insulin/Medications		
				Heart Rate (per min)	Type/Units	Pre	Post
Before:	Time:	(systolic):					
After:	Time:	(diastolic):					

Snack #2

Totals:								

Blood Glucose Levels		Blood Pressure Levels		Insulin/Medications		
				Heart Rate (per min)	Type/Units	Pre	Post
Before:	Time:	(systolic):					
After:	Time:	(diastolic):					

Dinner

Totals:								

Blood Glucose Levels		Blood Pressure Levels		Insulin/Medications		
				Heart Rate (per min)	Type/Units	Pre	Post
Before:	Time:	(systolic):					
After:	Time:	(diastolic):					

Fasting Blood Sugar:

_____

Water Intake:

total ounces _____

Fitness Log:

Activity	Min

Sleep Log:

Total Hours _____

Notes:

_____
_____
_____
_____
_____
_____
_____
_____
_____
_____

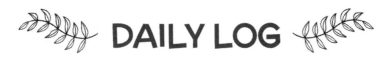

DAILY LOG

Date: ___/___/_____   **M T W Th F Sa Su**

Breakfast

Meal	Calories	Fat (g)	Carbs (g)	Sugar (g)	Fiber (g)	Net Carb (carbs-fiber)	Protein (g)	Sodium (mg)
Totals:								

Blood Glucose Levels			Blood Pressure Levels		Insulin/Medications		
Before:		Time:	(systolic):	Heart Rate (per min)	Type/Units	Pre	Post
After:		Time:	(diastolic):				

Snack #1

Totals:								

Blood Glucose Levels			Blood Pressure Levels		Insulin/Medications		
Before:		Time:	(systolic):	Heart Rate (per min)	Type/Units	Pre	Post
After:		Time:	(diastolic):				

Lunch

Totals:								

Blood Glucose Levels			Blood Pressure Levels		Insulin/Medications		
Before:		Time:	(systolic):	Heart Rate (per min)	Type/Units	Pre	Post
After:		Time:	(diastolic):				

Snack #2

Totals:								

Blood Glucose Levels			Blood Pressure Levels		Insulin/Medications		
Before:		Time:	(systolic):	Heart Rate (per min)	Type/Units	Pre	Post
After:		Time:	(diastolic):				

Dinner

Totals:								

Blood Glucose Levels			Blood Pressure Levels		Insulin/Medications		
Before:		Time:	(systolic):	Heart Rate (per min)	Type/Units	Pre	Post
After:		Time:	(diastolic):				

Fasting Blood Sugar:

_____

Water Intake:

total ounces _____

Fitness Log:

Activity	Min

Sleep Log:

Total Hours _____

Notes:

_____
_____
_____
_____
_____
_____
_____
_____

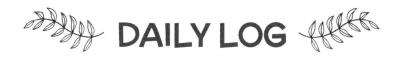

DAILY LOG

Date: ___/___/_____   **M T W Th F Sa Su**

Breakfast

	Meal	Calories	Fat (g)	Carbs (g)	Sugar (g)	Fiber (g)	Net Carb (carbs-fiber)	Protein (g)	Sodium (mg)
	Totals:								

Blood Glucose Levels			Blood Pressure Levels			Insulin/Medications		
					Heart Rate (per min)	Type/Units	Pre	Post
Before:		Time:	(systolic):					
After:		Time:	(diastolic):					

Snack #1

	Totals:								

Blood Glucose Levels			Blood Pressure Levels			Insulin/Medications		
					Heart Rate (per min)	Type/Units	Pre	Post
Before:		Time:	(systolic):					
After:		Time:	(diastolic):					

Lunch

	Totals:								

Blood Glucose Levels			Blood Pressure Levels			Insulin/Medications		
					Heart Rate (per min)	Type/Units	Pre	Post
Before:		Time:	(systolic):					
After:		Time:	(diastolic):					

Snack #2

	Totals:								

Blood Glucose Levels			Blood Pressure Levels			Insulin/Medications		
					Heart Rate (per min)	Type/Units	Pre	Post
Before:		Time:	(systolic):					
After:		Time:	(diastolic):					

Dinner

	Totals:								

Blood Glucose Levels			Blood Pressure Levels			Insulin/Medications		
					Heart Rate (per min)	Type/Units	Pre	Post
Before:		Time:	(systolic):					
After:		Time:	(diastolic):					

Fasting Blood Sugar:

_____

Water Intake:

total ounces _____

Fitness Log:

Activity	Min

Sleep Log:

Total Hours _____

Notes:

_____
_____
_____
_____
_____
_____
_____
_____

DAILY LOG
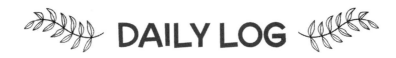

Date: ___/___/_____   **M   T   W   Th   F   Sa   Su**

Breakfast

Meal	Calories	Fat (g)	Carbs (g)	Sugar (g)	Fiber (g)	Net Carb (carbs-fiber)	Protein (g)	Sodium (mg)
Totals:								

Blood Glucose Levels			Blood Pressure Levels			Insulin/Medications		
Before:		Time:	(systolic):		Heart Rate (per min)	Type/Units	Pre	Post
After:		Time:	(diastolic):					

Snack #1

Meal	Calories	Fat (g)	Carbs (g)	Sugar (g)	Fiber (g)	Net Carb (carbs-fiber)	Protein (g)	Sodium (mg)
Totals:								

Blood Glucose Levels			Blood Pressure Levels			Insulin/Medications		
Before:		Time:	(systolic):		Heart Rate (per min)	Type/Units	Pre	Post
After:		Time:	(diastolic):					

Lunch

Meal	Calories	Fat (g)	Carbs (g)	Sugar (g)	Fiber (g)	Net Carb (carbs-fiber)	Protein (g)	Sodium (mg)
Totals:								

Blood Glucose Levels			Blood Pressure Levels			Insulin/Medications		
Before:		Time:	(systolic):		Heart Rate (per min)	Type/Units	Pre	Post
After:		Time:	(diastolic):					

Snack #2

Meal	Calories	Fat (g)	Carbs (g)	Sugar (g)	Fiber (g)	Net Carb (carbs-fiber)	Protein (g)	Sodium (mg)
Totals:								

Blood Glucose Levels			Blood Pressure Levels			Insulin/Medications		
Before:		Time:	(systolic):		Heart Rate (per min)	Type/Units	Pre	Post
After:		Time:	(diastolic):					

Dinner

Meal	Calories	Fat (g)	Carbs (g)	Sugar (g)	Fiber (g)	Net Carb (carbs-fiber)	Protein (g)	Sodium (mg)
Totals:								

Blood Glucose Levels			Blood Pressure Levels			Insulin/Medications		
Before:		Time:	(systolic):		Heart Rate (per min)	Type/Units	Pre	Post
After:		Time:	(diastolic):					

Fasting Blood Sugar:

_____

Water Intake:

total ounces _____

Fitness Log:

Activity		Min

Sleep Log:

Total Hours _____

Notes:

_____
_____
_____
_____
_____
_____
_____
_____
_____
_____
_____

DAILY LOG

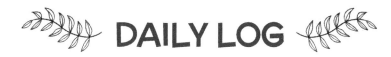

Date: ____/____/_____   **M T W Th F Sa Su**

Breakfast

Meal	Calories	Fat (g)	Carbs (g)	Sugar (g)	Fiber (g)	Net Carb (carbs-fiber)	Protein (g)	Sodium (mg)
Totals:								

Blood Glucose Levels			Blood Pressure Levels		Insulin/Medications		
Before:		Time:	(systolic):	Heart Rate (per min)	Type/Units	Pre	Post
After:		Time:	(diastolic):				

Snack #1

Totals:								

Blood Glucose Levels			Blood Pressure Levels		Insulin/Medications		
Before:		Time:	(systolic):	Heart Rate (per min)	Type/Units	Pre	Post
After:		Time:	(diastolic):				

Lunch

Totals:								

Blood Glucose Levels			Blood Pressure Levels		Insulin/Medications		
Before:		Time:	(systolic):	Heart Rate (per min)	Type/Units	Pre	Post
After:		Time:	(diastolic):				

Snack #2

Totals:								

Blood Glucose Levels			Blood Pressure Levels		Insulin/Medications		
Before:		Time:	(systolic):	Heart Rate (per min)	Type/Units	Pre	Post
After:		Time:	(diastolic):				

Dinner

Totals:								

Blood Glucose Levels			Blood Pressure Levels		Insulin/Medications		
Before:		Time:	(systolic):	Heart Rate (per min)	Type/Units	Pre	Post
After:		Time:	(diastolic):				

Fasting Blood Sugar:

_____

Water Intake:

🍶 🍶 🍶 🍶 🍶 🍶 🍶 🍶

total ounces _____

Fitness Log:

Activity	Min

Sleep Log:

Total Hours _____

Notes:

_____
_____
_____
_____
_____
_____
_____
_____
_____

DAILY LOG

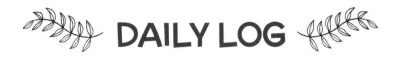

Date: ___/___/_____   **M T W Th F Sa Su**

Breakfast

Meal	Calories	Fat (g)	Carbs (g)	Sugar (g)	Fiber (g)	Net Carb (carbs-fiber)	Protein (g)	Sodium (mg)
Totals:								

Blood Glucose Levels			Blood Pressure Levels		Insulin/Medications		
Before:		Time:	(systolic):	Heart Rate (per min)	Type/Units	Pre	Post
After:		Time:	(diastolic):				

Snack #1

Totals:								

Blood Glucose Levels			Blood Pressure Levels		Insulin/Medications		
Before:		Time:	(systolic):	Heart Rate (per min)	Type/Units	Pre	Post
After:		Time:	(diastolic):				

Lunch

Totals:								

Blood Glucose Levels			Blood Pressure Levels		Insulin/Medications		
Before:		Time:	(systolic):	Heart Rate (per min)	Type/Units	Pre	Post
After:		Time:	(diastolic):				

Snack #2

Totals:								

Blood Glucose Levels			Blood Pressure Levels		Insulin/Medications		
Before:		Time:	(systolic):	Heart Rate (per min)	Type/Units	Pre	Post
After:		Time:	(diastolic):				

Dinner

Totals:								

Blood Glucose Levels			Blood Pressure Levels		Insulin/Medications		
Before:		Time:	(systolic):	Heart Rate (per min)	Type/Units	Pre	Post
After:		Time:	(diastolic):				

Fasting Blood Sugar:

_____

Water Intake:

🍼 🍼 🍼 🍼 🍼 🍼 🍼 🍼

total ounces _____

Fitness Log:

Activity   Min

Sleep Log:

Total Hours _____

Notes:

_____
_____
_____
_____
_____
_____
_____
_____
_____
_____

DAILY LOG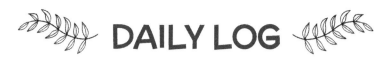

Date: ___/___/_____   **M T W Th F Sa Su**

Breakfast

	Meal	Calories	Fat (g)	Carbs (g)	Sugar (g)	Fiber (g)	Net Carb (carbs-fiber)	Protein (g)	Sodium (mg)
	Totals:								

Blood Glucose Levels				Blood Pressure Levels			Insulin/Medications		
Before:		Time:		(systolic):		Heart Rate (per min)	Type/Units	Pre	Post
After:		Time:		(diastolic):					

Fasting Blood Sugar:

_____

Snack #1

	Totals:								

Blood Glucose Levels				Blood Pressure Levels			Insulin/Medications		
Before:		Time:		(systolic):		Heart Rate (per min)	Type/Units	Pre	Post
After:		Time:		(diastolic):					

Water Intake:

total ounces _____

Fitness Log:

Activity	Min

Lunch

	Totals:								

Blood Glucose Levels				Blood Pressure Levels			Insulin/Medications		
Before:		Time:		(systolic):		Heart Rate (per min)	Type/Units	Pre	Post
After:		Time:		(diastolic):					

Sleep Log:

Total Hours _____

Snack #2

	Totals:								

Blood Glucose Levels				Blood Pressure Levels			Insulin/Medications		
Before:		Time:		(systolic):		Heart Rate (per min)	Type/Units	Pre	Post
After:		Time:		(diastolic):					

Notes:

_____
_____
_____

Dinner

	Totals:								

Blood Glucose Levels				Blood Pressure Levels			Insulin/Medications		
Before:		Time:		(systolic):		Heart Rate (per min)	Type/Units	Pre	Post
After:		Time:		(diastolic):					

DAILY LOG

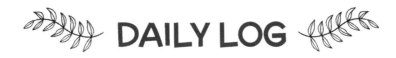

Date: ___/___/_____   M T W Th F Sa Su

Breakfast

Meal	Calories	Fat (g)	Carbs (g)	Sugar (g)	Fiber (g)	Net Carb (carbs-fiber)	Protein (g)	Sodium (mg)
Totals:								

Blood Glucose Levels			Blood Pressure Levels			Insulin/Medications		
Before:		Time:	(systolic):		Heart Rate (per min)	Type/Units	Pre	Post
After:		Time:	(diastolic):					

Snack #1

Meal	Calories	Fat (g)	Carbs (g)	Sugar (g)	Fiber (g)	Net Carb (carbs-fiber)	Protein (g)	Sodium (mg)
Totals:								

Blood Glucose Levels			Blood Pressure Levels			Insulin/Medications		
Before:		Time:	(systolic):		Heart Rate (per min)	Type/Units	Pre	Post
After:		Time:	(diastolic):					

Lunch

Meal	Calories	Fat (g)	Carbs (g)	Sugar (g)	Fiber (g)	Net Carb (carbs-fiber)	Protein (g)	Sodium (mg)
Totals:								

Blood Glucose Levels			Blood Pressure Levels			Insulin/Medications		
Before:		Time:	(systolic):		Heart Rate (per min)	Type/Units	Pre	Post
After:		Time:	(diastolic):					

Snack #2

Meal	Calories	Fat (g)	Carbs (g)	Sugar (g)	Fiber (g)	Net Carb (carbs-fiber)	Protein (g)	Sodium (mg)
Totals:								

Blood Glucose Levels			Blood Pressure Levels			Insulin/Medications		
Before:		Time:	(systolic):		Heart Rate (per min)	Type/Units	Pre	Post
After:		Time:	(diastolic):					

Dinner

Meal	Calories	Fat (g)	Carbs (g)	Sugar (g)	Fiber (g)	Net Carb (carbs-fiber)	Protein (g)	Sodium (mg)
Totals:								

Blood Glucose Levels			Blood Pressure Levels			Insulin/Medications		
Before:		Time:	(systolic):		Heart Rate (per min)	Type/Units	Pre	Post
After:		Time:	(diastolic):					

Fasting Blood Sugar:

_____

Water Intake:

total ounces _____

Fitness Log:

Activity	Min

Sleep Log:

Total Hours _____

Notes:

_____
_____
_____
_____
_____
_____
_____
_____
_____

DAILY LOG

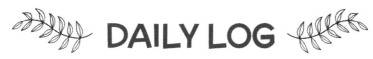

Date: ___/___/_____   **M T W Th F Sa Su**

Breakfast

Meal	Calories	Fat (g)	Carbs (g)	Sugar (g)	Fiber (g)	Net Carb (carbs-fiber)	Protein (g)	Sodium (mg)
Totals:								

Blood Glucose Levels		Blood Pressure Levels		Insulin/Medications		
			Heart Rate (per min)	Type/Units	Pre	Post
Before:	Time:	(systolic):				
After:	Time:	(diastolic):				

Snack #1

Totals:								

Blood Glucose Levels		Blood Pressure Levels		Insulin/Medications		
			Heart Rate (per min)	Type/Units	Pre	Post
Before:	Time:	(systolic):				
After:	Time:	(diastolic):				

Lunch

Totals:								

Blood Glucose Levels		Blood Pressure Levels		Insulin/Medications		
			Heart Rate (per min)	Type/Units	Pre	Post
Before:	Time:	(systolic):				
After:	Time:	(diastolic):				

Snack #2

Totals:								

Blood Glucose Levels		Blood Pressure Levels		Insulin/Medications		
			Heart Rate (per min)	Type/Units	Pre	Post
Before:	Time:	(systolic):				
After:	Time:	(diastolic):				

Dinner

Totals:								

Blood Glucose Levels		Blood Pressure Levels		Insulin/Medications		
			Heart Rate (per min)	Type/Units	Pre	Post
Before:	Time:	(systolic):				
After:	Time:	(diastolic):				

Fasting Blood Sugar:

_____

Water Intake:

total ounces _____

Fitness Log:

Activity	Min

Sleep Log:

Total Hours _____

Notes:

_____
_____
_____
_____
_____
_____
_____
_____
_____

DAILY LOG

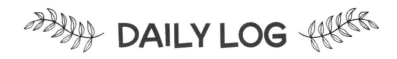

Date: ___/___/_____   **M T W Th F Sa Su**

Breakfast

	Meal	Calories	Fat (g)	Carbs (g)	Sugar (g)	Fiber (g)	Net Carb (carbs-fiber)	Protein (g)	Sodium (mg)
	Totals:								

Blood Glucose Levels				Blood Pressure Levels			Insulin/Medications		
Before:		Time:		(systolic):		Heart Rate (per min)	Type/Units	Pre	Post
After:		Time:		(diastolic):					

Snack #1

	Totals:								

Blood Glucose Levels				Blood Pressure Levels			Insulin/Medications		
Before:		Time:		(systolic):		Heart Rate (per min)	Type/Units	Pre	Post
After:		Time:		(diastolic):					

Lunch

	Totals:								

Blood Glucose Levels				Blood Pressure Levels			Insulin/Medications		
Before:		Time:		(systolic):		Heart Rate (per min)	Type/Units	Pre	Post
After:		Time:		(diastolic):					

Snack #2

	Totals:								

Blood Glucose Levels				Blood Pressure Levels			Insulin/Medications		
Before:		Time:		(systolic):		Heart Rate (per min)	Type/Units	Pre	Post
After:		Time:		(diastolic):					

Dinner

	Totals:								

Blood Glucose Levels				Blood Pressure Levels			Insulin/Medications		
Before:		Time:		(systolic):		Heart Rate (per min)	Type/Units	Pre	Post
After:		Time:		(diastolic):					

Fasting Blood Sugar:
_____

Water Intake:
total ounces _____

Fitness Log:
Activity   Min

Sleep Log:
Total Hours _____

Notes:

DAILY LOG

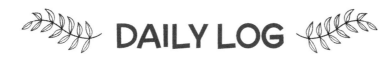

Date: ___/___/_____   **M   T   W   Th   F   Sa   Su**

Breakfast

	Meal	Calories	Fat (g)	Carbs (g)	Sugar (g)	Fiber (g)	Net Carb (carbs-fiber)	Protein (g)	Sodium (mg)
	Totals:								

Blood Glucose Levels			Blood Pressure Levels		Insulin/Medications		
Before:		Time:	(systolic):	Heart Rate (per min)	Type/Units	Pre	Post
After:		Time:	(diastolic):				

Snack #1

	Totals:								

Blood Glucose Levels			Blood Pressure Levels		Insulin/Medications		
Before:		Time:	(systolic):	Heart Rate (per min)	Type/Units	Pre	Post
After:		Time:	(diastolic):				

Lunch

	Totals:								

Blood Glucose Levels			Blood Pressure Levels		Insulin/Medications		
Before:		Time:	(systolic):	Heart Rate (per min)	Type/Units	Pre	Post
After:		Time:	(diastolic):				

Snack #2

	Totals:								

Blood Glucose Levels			Blood Pressure Levels		Insulin/Medications		
Before:		Time:	(systolic):	Heart Rate (per min)	Type/Units	Pre	Post
After:		Time:	(diastolic):				

Dinner

	Totals:								

Blood Glucose Levels			Blood Pressure Levels		Insulin/Medications		
Before:		Time:	(systolic):	Heart Rate (per min)	Type/Units	Pre	Post
After:		Time:	(diastolic):				

Fasting Blood Sugar:

_____

Water Intake:

total ounces _____

Fitness Log:

Activity	Min

Sleep Log:

Total Hours _____

Notes:

DAILY LOG
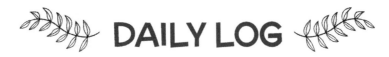

Date: ___/___/_____   **M T W Th F Sa Su**

Breakfast

Meal	Calories	Fat (g)	Carbs (g)	Sugar (g)	Fiber (g)	Net Carb (carbs-fiber)	Protein (g)	Sodium (mg)
Totals:								

Blood Glucose Levels			Blood Pressure Levels			Insulin/Medications		
Before:		Time:	(systolic):		Heart Rate (per min)	Type/Units	Pre	Post
After:		Time:	(diastolic):					

Snack #1

Totals:								

Blood Glucose Levels			Blood Pressure Levels			Insulin/Medications		
Before:		Time:	(systolic):		Heart Rate (per min)	Type/Units	Pre	Post
After:		Time:	(diastolic):					

Lunch

Totals:								

Blood Glucose Levels			Blood Pressure Levels			Insulin/Medications		
Before:		Time:	(systolic):		Heart Rate (per min)	Type/Units	Pre	Post
After:		Time:	(diastolic):					

Snack #2

Totals:								

Blood Glucose Levels			Blood Pressure Levels			Insulin/Medications		
Before:		Time:	(systolic):		Heart Rate (per min)	Type/Units	Pre	Post
After:		Time:	(diastolic):					

Dinner

Totals:								

Blood Glucose Levels			Blood Pressure Levels			Insulin/Medications		
Before:		Time:	(systolic):		Heart Rate (per min)	Type/Units	Pre	Post
After:		Time:	(diastolic):					

Fasting Blood Sugar:
_____

Water Intake:
total ounces _____

Fitness Log:

Activity	Min

Sleep Log:
Total Hours _____

Notes:
_____
_____
_____
_____
_____
_____
_____

DAILY LOG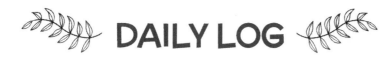

Date: ___/___/_____   **M T W Th F Sa Su**

Breakfast

Meal	Calories	Fat (g)	Carbs (g)	Sugar (g)	Fiber (g)	Net Carb (carbs-fiber)	Protein (g)	Sodium (mg)
Totals:								

Blood Glucose Levels			Blood Pressure Levels			Insulin/Medications		
Before:		Time:	(systolic):		Heart Rate (per min)	Type/Units	Pre	Post
After:		Time:	(diastolic):					

Snack #1

Totals:								

Blood Glucose Levels			Blood Pressure Levels			Insulin/Medications		
Before:		Time:	(systolic):		Heart Rate (per min)	Type/Units	Pre	Post
After:		Time:	(diastolic):					

Lunch

Totals:								

Blood Glucose Levels			Blood Pressure Levels			Insulin/Medications		
Before:		Time:	(systolic):		Heart Rate (per min)	Type/Units	Pre	Post
After:		Time:	(diastolic):					

Snack #2

Totals:								

Blood Glucose Levels			Blood Pressure Levels			Insulin/Medications		
Before:		Time:	(systolic):		Heart Rate (per min)	Type/Units	Pre	Post
After:		Time:	(diastolic):					

Dinner

Totals:								

Blood Glucose Levels			Blood Pressure Levels			Insulin/Medications		
Before:		Time:	(systolic):		Heart Rate (per min)	Type/Units	Pre	Post
After:		Time:	(diastolic):					

Fasting Blood Sugar:

_____

Water Intake:

total ounces _____

Fitness Log:

Activity	Min

Sleep Log:

Total Hours _____

Notes:

_____
_____
_____
_____
_____
_____
_____
_____

DAILY LOG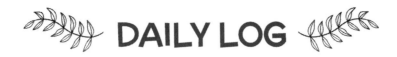

Date: ___/___/_____   **M T W Th F Sa Su**

Breakfast

Meal	Calories	Fat (g)	Carbs (g)	Sugar (g)	Fiber (g)	Net Carb (carbs-fiber)	Protein (g)	Sodium (mg)
Totals:								

Blood Glucose Levels			Blood Pressure Levels			Insulin/Medications		
Before:		Time:		(systolic):	Heart Rate (per min)	Type/Units	Pre	Post
After:		Time:		(diastolic):				

Snack #1

Meal	Calories	Fat (g)	Carbs (g)	Sugar (g)	Fiber (g)	Net Carb (carbs-fiber)	Protein (g)	Sodium (mg)
Totals:								

Blood Glucose Levels			Blood Pressure Levels			Insulin/Medications		
Before:		Time:		(systolic):	Heart Rate (per min)	Type/Units	Pre	Post
After:		Time:		(diastolic):				

Lunch

Meal	Calories	Fat (g)	Carbs (g)	Sugar (g)	Fiber (g)	Net Carb (carbs-fiber)	Protein (g)	Sodium (mg)
Totals:								

Blood Glucose Levels			Blood Pressure Levels			Insulin/Medications		
Before:		Time:		(systolic):	Heart Rate (per min)	Type/Units	Pre	Post
After:		Time:		(diastolic):				

Snack #2

Meal	Calories	Fat (g)	Carbs (g)	Sugar (g)	Fiber (g)	Net Carb (carbs-fiber)	Protein (g)	Sodium (mg)
Totals:								

Blood Glucose Levels			Blood Pressure Levels			Insulin/Medications		
Before:		Time:		(systolic):	Heart Rate (per min)	Type/Units	Pre	Post
After:		Time:		(diastolic):				

Dinner

Meal	Calories	Fat (g)	Carbs (g)	Sugar (g)	Fiber (g)	Net Carb (carbs-fiber)	Protein (g)	Sodium (mg)
Totals:								

Blood Glucose Levels			Blood Pressure Levels			Insulin/Medications		
Before:		Time:		(systolic):	Heart Rate (per min)	Type/Units	Pre	Post
After:		Time:		(diastolic):				

Fasting Blood Sugar:

_____

Water Intake:

total ounces _____

Fitness Log:

Activity	Min

Sleep Log:

Total Hours _____

Notes:

DAILY LOG

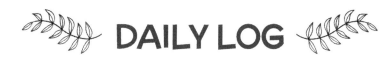

Date: ___/___/_____   **M T W Th F Sa Su**

Breakfast

Meal	Calories	Fat (g)	Carbs (g)	Sugar (g)	Fiber (g)	Net Carb (carbs-fiber)	Protein (g)	Sodium (mg)
Totals:								

Blood Glucose Levels			Blood Pressure Levels			Insulin/Medications		
Before:		Time:	(systolic):		Heart Rate (per min)	Type/Units	Pre	Post
After:		Time:	(diastolic):					

Snack #1

Totals:								

Blood Glucose Levels			Blood Pressure Levels			Insulin/Medications		
Before:		Time:	(systolic):		Heart Rate (per min)	Type/Units	Pre	Post
After:		Time:	(diastolic):					

Lunch

Totals:								

Blood Glucose Levels			Blood Pressure Levels			Insulin/Medications		
Before:		Time:	(systolic):		Heart Rate (per min)	Type/Units	Pre	Post
After:		Time:	(diastolic):					

Snack #2

Totals:								

Blood Glucose Levels			Blood Pressure Levels			Insulin/Medications		
Before:		Time:	(systolic):		Heart Rate (per min)	Type/Units	Pre	Post
After:		Time:	(diastolic):					

Dinner

Totals:								

Blood Glucose Levels			Blood Pressure Levels			Insulin/Medications		
Before:		Time:	(systolic):		Heart Rate (per min)	Type/Units	Pre	Post
After:		Time:	(diastolic):					

Fasting Blood Sugar:

_____

Water Intake:

total ounces _____

Fitness Log:

Activity	Min

Sleep Log:

Total Hours _____

Notes:

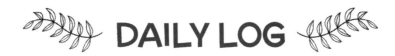

DAILY LOG

Date: ____/____/_____   **M   T   W   Th   F   Sa   Su**

Breakfast

Meal	Calories	Fat (g)	Carbs (g)	Sugar (g)	Fiber (g)	Net Carb (carbs-fiber)	Protein (g)	Sodium (mg)
Totals:								

Blood Glucose Levels				Blood Pressure Levels			Insulin/Medications		
Before:		Time:		(systolic):		Heart Rate (per min)	Type/Units	Pre	Post
After:		Time:		(diastolic):					

Snack #1

Meal	Calories	Fat (g)	Carbs (g)	Sugar (g)	Fiber (g)	Net Carb (carbs-fiber)	Protein (g)	Sodium (mg)
Totals:								

Blood Glucose Levels				Blood Pressure Levels			Insulin/Medications		
Before:		Time:		(systolic):		Heart Rate (per min)	Type/Units	Pre	Post
After:		Time:		(diastolic):					

Lunch

Meal	Calories	Fat (g)	Carbs (g)	Sugar (g)	Fiber (g)	Net Carb (carbs-fiber)	Protein (g)	Sodium (mg)
Totals:								

Blood Glucose Levels				Blood Pressure Levels			Insulin/Medications		
Before:		Time:		(systolic):		Heart Rate (per min)	Type/Units	Pre	Post
After:		Time:		(diastolic):					

Snack #2

Meal	Calories	Fat (g)	Carbs (g)	Sugar (g)	Fiber (g)	Net Carb (carbs-fiber)	Protein (g)	Sodium (mg)
Totals:								

Blood Glucose Levels				Blood Pressure Levels			Insulin/Medications		
Before:		Time:		(systolic):		Heart Rate (per min)	Type/Units	Pre	Post
After:		Time:		(diastolic):					

Dinner

Meal	Calories	Fat (g)	Carbs (g)	Sugar (g)	Fiber (g)	Net Carb (carbs-fiber)	Protein (g)	Sodium (mg)
Totals:								

Blood Glucose Levels				Blood Pressure Levels			Insulin/Medications		
Before:		Time:		(systolic):		Heart Rate (per min)	Type/Units	Pre	Post
After:		Time:		(diastolic):					

Fasting Blood Sugar:

_____

Water Intake:

total ounces _____

Fitness Log:

Activity	Min

Sleep Log:

Total Hours _____

Notes:

DAILY LOG

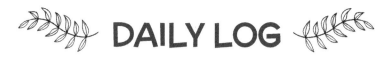

Date: ___/___/_____   M T W Th F Sa Su

Breakfast

	Meal	Calories	Fat (g)	Carbs (g)	Sugar (g)	Fiber (g)	Net Carb (carbs-fiber)	Protein (g)	Sodium (mg)
	Totals:								

Blood Glucose Levels			Blood Pressure Levels			Insulin/Medications		
Before:		Time:	(systolic):		Heart Rate (per min)	Type/Units	Pre	Post
After:		Time:	(diastolic):					

Snack #1

	Totals:								

Blood Glucose Levels			Blood Pressure Levels			Insulin/Medications		
Before:		Time:	(systolic):		Heart Rate (per min)	Type/Units	Pre	Post
After:		Time:	(diastolic):					

Lunch

	Totals:								

Blood Glucose Levels			Blood Pressure Levels			Insulin/Medications		
Before:		Time:	(systolic):		Heart Rate (per min)	Type/Units	Pre	Post
After:		Time:	(diastolic):					

Snack #2

	Totals:								

Blood Glucose Levels			Blood Pressure Levels			Insulin/Medications		
Before:		Time:	(systolic):		Heart Rate (per min)	Type/Units	Pre	Post
After:		Time:	(diastolic):					

Dinner

	Totals:								

Blood Glucose Levels			Blood Pressure Levels			Insulin/Medications		
Before:		Time:	(systolic):		Heart Rate (per min)	Type/Units	Pre	Post
After:		Time:	(diastolic):					

Fasting Blood Sugar:
_____

Water Intake:
total ounces _____

Fitness Log:
Activity   Min

Sleep Log:
Total Hours _____

Notes:

DAILY LOG
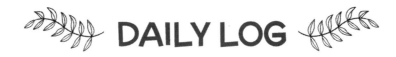

Date: ___/___/_____   **M   T   W   Th   F   Sa   Su**

Breakfast

Meal	Calories	Fat (g)	Carbs (g)	Sugar (g)	Fiber (g)	Net Carb (carbs-fiber)	Protein (g)	Sodium (mg)
Totals:								

Blood Glucose Levels				Blood Pressure Levels			Insulin/Medications		
Before:		Time:		(systolic):		Heart Rate (per min)	Type/Units	Pre	Post
After:		Time:		(diastolic):					

Snack #1

Totals:								

Blood Glucose Levels				Blood Pressure Levels			Insulin/Medications		
Before:		Time:		(systolic):		Heart Rate (per min)	Type/Units	Pre	Post
After:		Time:		(diastolic):					

Lunch

Totals:								

Blood Glucose Levels				Blood Pressure Levels			Insulin/Medications		
Before:		Time:		(systolic):		Heart Rate (per min)	Type/Units	Pre	Post
After:		Time:		(diastolic):					

Snack #2

Totals:								

Blood Glucose Levels				Blood Pressure Levels			Insulin/Medications		
Before:		Time:		(systolic):		Heart Rate (per min)	Type/Units	Pre	Post
After:		Time:		(diastolic):					

Dinner

Totals:								

Blood Glucose Levels				Blood Pressure Levels			Insulin/Medications		
Before:		Time:		(systolic):		Heart Rate (per min)	Type/Units	Pre	Post
After:		Time:		(diastolic):					

Fasting Blood Sugar:
_____

Water Intake:
total ounces _____

Fitness Log:

Activity	Min

Sleep Log:
Total Hours _____

Notes:
_____
_____
_____
_____
_____
_____
_____
_____
_____
_____

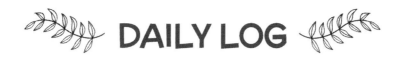

DAILY LOG

Date: ___/___/_____   **M T W Th F Sa Su**

Breakfast

Meal	Calories	Fat (g)	Carbs (g)	Sugar (g)	Fiber (g)	Net Carb (carbs-fiber)	Protein (g)	Sodium (mg)
Totals:								

Blood Glucose Levels			Blood Pressure Levels			Insulin/Medications		
Before:		Time:	(systolic):		Heart Rate (per min)	Type/Units	Pre	Post
After:		Time:	(diastolic):					

Snack #1

Totals:								

Blood Glucose Levels			Blood Pressure Levels			Insulin/Medications		
Before:		Time:	(systolic):		Heart Rate (per min)	Type/Units	Pre	Post
After:		Time:	(diastolic):					

Lunch

Totals:								

Blood Glucose Levels			Blood Pressure Levels			Insulin/Medications		
Before:		Time:	(systolic):		Heart Rate (per min)	Type/Units	Pre	Post
After:		Time:	(diastolic):					

Snack #2

Totals:								

Blood Glucose Levels			Blood Pressure Levels			Insulin/Medications		
Before:		Time:	(systolic):		Heart Rate (per min)	Type/Units	Pre	Post
After:		Time:	(diastolic):					

Dinner

Totals:								

Blood Glucose Levels			Blood Pressure Levels			Insulin/Medications		
Before:		Time:	(systolic):		Heart Rate (per min)	Type/Units	Pre	Post
After:		Time:	(diastolic):					

Fasting Blood Sugar:
_____

Water Intake:
total ounces _____

Fitness Log:

Activity	Min

Sleep Log:
Total Hours _____

Notes:

DAILY LOG
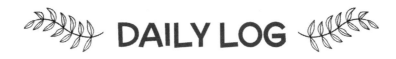

Date: ___/___/_____   **M T W Th F Sa Su**

Breakfast

Meal	Calories	Fat (g)	Carbs (g)	Sugar (g)	Fiber (g)	Net Carb (carbs-fiber)	Protein (g)	Sodium (mg)
Totals:								

Blood Glucose Levels			Blood Pressure Levels			Insulin/Medications		
Before:		Time:	(systolic):		Heart Rate (per min)	Type/Units	Pre	Post
After:		Time:	(diastolic):					

Snack #1

Totals:								

Blood Glucose Levels			Blood Pressure Levels			Insulin/Medications		
Before:		Time:	(systolic):		Heart Rate (per min)	Type/Units	Pre	Post
After:		Time:	(diastolic):					

Lunch

Totals:								

Blood Glucose Levels			Blood Pressure Levels			Insulin/Medications		
Before:		Time:	(systolic):		Heart Rate (per min)	Type/Units	Pre	Post
After:		Time:	(diastolic):					

Snack #2

Totals:								

Blood Glucose Levels			Blood Pressure Levels			Insulin/Medications		
Before:		Time:	(systolic):		Heart Rate (per min)	Type/Units	Pre	Post
After:		Time:	(diastolic):					

Dinner

Totals:								

Blood Glucose Levels			Blood Pressure Levels			Insulin/Medications		
Before:		Time:	(systolic):		Heart Rate (per min)	Type/Units	Pre	Post
After:		Time:	(diastolic):					

Fasting Blood Sugar:

_____

Water Intake:

total ounces _____

Fitness Log:

Activity	Min

Sleep Log:

Total Hours _____

Notes:

_____
_____
_____
_____
_____
_____
_____
_____

DAILY LOG

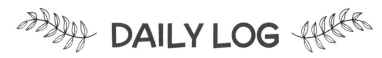

Date: ___/___/_____   **M T W Th F Sa Su**

Breakfast

Meal	Calories	Fat (g)	Carbs (g)	Sugar (g)	Fiber (g)	Net Carb (carbs-fiber)	Protein (g)	Sodium (mg)
Totals:								

Blood Glucose Levels			Blood Pressure Levels			Insulin/Medications		
Before:		Time:	(systolic):		Heart Rate (per min)	Type/Units	Pre	Post
After:		Time:	(diastolic):					

Snack #1

Totals:								

Blood Glucose Levels			Blood Pressure Levels			Insulin/Medications		
Before:		Time:	(systolic):		Heart Rate (per min)	Type/Units	Pre	Post
After:		Time:	(diastolic):					

Lunch

Totals:								

Blood Glucose Levels			Blood Pressure Levels			Insulin/Medications		
Before:		Time:	(systolic):		Heart Rate (per min)	Type/Units	Pre	Post
After:		Time:	(diastolic):					

Snack #2

Totals:								

Blood Glucose Levels			Blood Pressure Levels			Insulin/Medications		
Before:		Time:	(systolic):		Heart Rate (per min)	Type/Units	Pre	Post
After:		Time:	(diastolic):					

Dinner

Totals:								

Blood Glucose Levels			Blood Pressure Levels			Insulin/Medications		
Before:		Time:	(systolic):		Heart Rate (per min)	Type/Units	Pre	Post
After:		Time:	(diastolic):					

Fasting Blood Sugar:

_____

Water Intake:

total ounces _____

Fitness Log:

Activity	Min

Sleep Log:

Total Hours _____

Notes:

_____
_____
_____
_____
_____
_____
_____
_____
_____

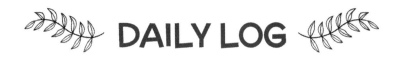

DAILY LOG

Date: ___/___/_____   **M T W Th F Sa Su**

Breakfast

Meal	Calories	Fat (g)	Carbs (g)	Sugar (g)	Fiber (g)	Net Carb (carbs-fiber)	Protein (g)	Sodium (mg)
Totals:								

Blood Glucose Levels			Blood Pressure Levels			Insulin/Medications		
Before:		Time:	(systolic):		Heart Rate (per min)	Type/Units	Pre	Post
After:		Time:	(diastolic):					

Snack #1

Totals:								

Blood Glucose Levels			Blood Pressure Levels			Insulin/Medications		
Before:		Time:	(systolic):		Heart Rate (per min)	Type/Units	Pre	Post
After:		Time:	(diastolic):					

Lunch

Totals:								

Blood Glucose Levels			Blood Pressure Levels			Insulin/Medications		
Before:		Time:	(systolic):		Heart Rate (per min)	Type/Units	Pre	Post
After:		Time:	(diastolic):					

Snack #2

Totals:								

Blood Glucose Levels			Blood Pressure Levels			Insulin/Medications		
Before:		Time:	(systolic):		Heart Rate (per min)	Type/Units	Pre	Post
After:		Time:	(diastolic):					

Dinner

Totals:								

Blood Glucose Levels			Blood Pressure Levels			Insulin/Medications		
Before:		Time:	(systolic):		Heart Rate (per min)	Type/Units	Pre	Post
After:		Time:	(diastolic):					

Fasting Blood Sugar:

_____

Water Intake:

total ounces _____

Fitness Log:

Activity	Min

Sleep Log:

Total Hours _____

Notes:

DAILY LOG

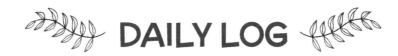

Date: ___/___/_____   **M T W Th F Sa Su**

Breakfast

	Meal	Calories	Fat (g)	Carbs (g)	Sugar (g)	Fiber (g)	Net Carb (carbs-fiber)	Protein (g)	Sodium (mg)
	Totals:								

Blood Glucose Levels			Blood Pressure Levels			Insulin/Medications		
Before:		Time:	(systolic):		Heart Rate (per min)	Type/Units	Pre	Post
After:		Time:	(diastolic):					

Fasting Blood Sugar:
_____

Water Intake:
total ounces _____

Snack #1

	Totals:								

Blood Glucose Levels			Blood Pressure Levels			Insulin/Medications		
Before:		Time:	(systolic):		Heart Rate (per min)	Type/Units	Pre	Post
After:		Time:	(diastolic):					

Fitness Log:

Activity	Min

Lunch

	Totals:								

Blood Glucose Levels			Blood Pressure Levels			Insulin/Medications		
Before:		Time:	(systolic):		Heart Rate (per min)	Type/Units	Pre	Post
After:		Time:	(diastolic):					

Sleep Log:
Total Hours _____

Snack #2

	Totals:								

Blood Glucose Levels			Blood Pressure Levels			Insulin/Medications		
Before:		Time:	(systolic):		Heart Rate (per min)	Type/Units	Pre	Post
After:		Time:	(diastolic):					

Notes:

Dinner

	Totals:								

Blood Glucose Levels			Blood Pressure Levels			Insulin/Medications		
Before:		Time:	(systolic):		Heart Rate (per min)	Type/Units	Pre	Post
After:		Time:	(diastolic):					

DAILY LOG

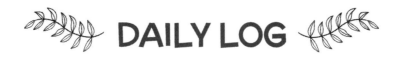

Date: ___/___/_____   **M T W Th F Sa Su**

Breakfast

Meal	Calories	Fat (g)	Carbs (g)	Sugar (g)	Fiber (g)	Net Carb (carbs-fiber)	Protein (g)	Sodium (mg)
Totals:								

Blood Glucose Levels				Blood Pressure Levels		Insulin/Medications		
Before:		Time:		(systolic):	Heart Rate (per min)	Type/Units	Pre	Post
After:		Time:		(diastolic):				

Snack #1

Meal	Calories	Fat (g)	Carbs (g)	Sugar (g)	Fiber (g)	Net Carb (carbs-fiber)	Protein (g)	Sodium (mg)
Totals:								

Blood Glucose Levels				Blood Pressure Levels		Insulin/Medications		
Before:		Time:		(systolic):	Heart Rate (per min)	Type/Units	Pre	Post
After:		Time:		(diastolic):				

Lunch

Meal	Calories	Fat (g)	Carbs (g)	Sugar (g)	Fiber (g)	Net Carb (carbs-fiber)	Protein (g)	Sodium (mg)
Totals:								

Blood Glucose Levels				Blood Pressure Levels		Insulin/Medications		
Before:		Time:		(systolic):	Heart Rate (per min)	Type/Units	Pre	Post
After:		Time:		(diastolic):				

Snack #2

Meal	Calories	Fat (g)	Carbs (g)	Sugar (g)	Fiber (g)	Net Carb (carbs-fiber)	Protein (g)	Sodium (mg)
Totals:								

Blood Glucose Levels				Blood Pressure Levels		Insulin/Medications		
Before:		Time:		(systolic):	Heart Rate (per min)	Type/Units	Pre	Post
After:		Time:		(diastolic):				

Dinner

Meal	Calories	Fat (g)	Carbs (g)	Sugar (g)	Fiber (g)	Net Carb (carbs-fiber)	Protein (g)	Sodium (mg)
Totals:								

Blood Glucose Levels				Blood Pressure Levels		Insulin/Medications		
Before:		Time:		(systolic):	Heart Rate (per min)	Type/Units	Pre	Post
After:		Time:		(diastolic):				

Fasting Blood Sugar:

_____

Water Intake:

🍶 🍶 🍶 🍶 🍶 🍶 🍶 🍶

total ounces _____

Fitness Log:

Activity	Min

Sleep Log:

Total Hours _____

Notes:

_____

_____

_____

_____

_____

_____

_____

_____

_____

_____

_____

DAILY LOG

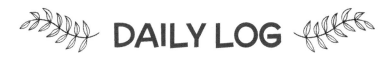

Date: ___/___/_____   **M T W Th F Sa Su**

Breakfast

	Meal	Calories	Fat (g)	Carbs (g)	Sugar (g)	Fiber (g)	Net Carb (carbs-fiber)	Protein (g)	Sodium (mg)
	Totals:								

Blood Glucose Levels			Blood Pressure Levels			Insulin/Medications		
Before:		Time:	(systolic):		Heart Rate (per min)	Type/Units	Pre	Post
After:		Time:	(diastolic):					

Snack #1

	Totals:								

Blood Glucose Levels			Blood Pressure Levels			Insulin/Medications		
Before:		Time:	(systolic):		Heart Rate (per min)	Type/Units	Pre	Post
After:		Time:	(diastolic):					

Lunch

	Totals:								

Blood Glucose Levels			Blood Pressure Levels			Insulin/Medications		
Before:		Time:	(systolic):		Heart Rate (per min)	Type/Units	Pre	Post
After:		Time:	(diastolic):					

Snack #2

	Totals:								

Blood Glucose Levels			Blood Pressure Levels			Insulin/Medications		
Before:		Time:	(systolic):		Heart Rate (per min)	Type/Units	Pre	Post
After:		Time:	(diastolic):					

Dinner

	Totals:								

Blood Glucose Levels			Blood Pressure Levels			Insulin/Medications		
Before:		Time:	(systolic):		Heart Rate (per min)	Type/Units	Pre	Post
After:		Time:	(diastolic):					

Fasting Blood Sugar:
_____

Water Intake:
total ounces _____

Fitness Log:
Activity   Min

Sleep Log:
Total Hours _____

Notes:

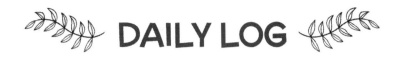

DAILY LOG

Date: ___/___/_____

M T W Th F Sa Su

Breakfast

Meal	Calories	Fat (g)	Carbs (g)	Sugar (g)	Fiber (g)	Net Corb (carbs-fiber)	Protein (g)	Sodium (mg)
Totals:								

Blood Glucose Levels			Blood Pressure Levels			Insulin/Medications		
Before:		Time:	(systolic):		Heart Rate (per min)	Type/Units	Pre	Post
After:		Time:	(diastolic):					

Snack #1

Totals:								

Blood Glucose Levels			Blood Pressure Levels			Insulin/Medications		
Before:		Time:	(systolic):		Heart Rate (per min)	Type/Units	Pre	Post
After:		Time:	(diastolic):					

Lunch

Totals:								

Blood Glucose Levels			Blood Pressure Levels			Insulin/Medications		
Before:		Time:	(systolic):		Heart Rate (per min)	Type/Units	Pre	Post
After:		Time:	(diastolic):					

Snack #2

Totals:								

Blood Glucose Levels			Blood Pressure Levels			Insulin/Medications		
Before:		Time:	(systolic):		Heart Rate (per min)	Type/Units	Pre	Post
After:		Time:	(diastolic):					

Dinner

Totals:								

Blood Glucose Levels			Blood Pressure Levels			Insulin/Medications		
Before:		Time:	(systolic):		Heart Rate (per min)	Type/Units	Pre	Post
After:		Time:	(diastolic):					

Fasting Blood Sugar:

_____

Water Intake:

total ounces _____

Fitness Log:

Activity	Min

Sleep Log:

Total Hours _____

Notes:

_____
_____
_____
_____
_____
_____
_____
_____
_____
_____

DAILY LOG

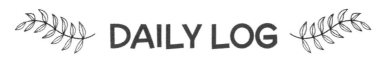

Date: ____/____/_____   **M T W Th F Sa Su**

Breakfast

	Meal	Calories	Fat (g)	Carbs (g)	Sugar (g)	Fiber (g)	Net Carb (carbs-fiber)	Protein (g)	Sodium (mg)
	Totals:								

Blood Glucose Levels			Blood Pressure Levels			Insulin/Medications		
Before:		Time:	(systolic):		Heart Rate (per min)	Type/Units	Pre	Post
After:		Time:	(diastolic):					

Snack #1

	Totals:								

Blood Glucose Levels			Blood Pressure Levels			Insulin/Medications		
Before:		Time:	(systolic):		Heart Rate (per min)	Type/Units	Pre	Post
After:		Time:	(diastolic):					

Lunch

	Totals:								

Blood Glucose Levels			Blood Pressure Levels			Insulin/Medications		
Before:		Time:	(systolic):		Heart Rate (per min)	Type/Units	Pre	Post
After:		Time:	(diastolic):					

Snack #2

	Totals:								

Blood Glucose Levels			Blood Pressure Levels			Insulin/Medications		
Before:		Time:	(systolic):		Heart Rate (per min)	Type/Units	Pre	Post
After:		Time:	(diastolic):					

Dinner

	Totals:								

Blood Glucose Levels			Blood Pressure Levels			Insulin/Medications		
Before:		Time:	(systolic):		Heart Rate (per min)	Type/Units	Pre	Post
After:		Time:	(diastolic):					

Fasting Blood Sugar:

_____

Water Intake:

total
ounces _____

Fitness Log:

Activity	Min

Sleep Log:

Total
Hours _____

Notes:

DAILY LOG

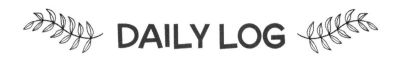

Date: ___/___/_____   **M T W Th F Sa Su**

Breakfast

Meal	Calories	Fat (g)	Carbs (g)	Sugar (g)	Fiber (g)	Net Carb (carbs-fiber)	Protein (g)	Sodium (mg)
Totals:								

Blood Glucose Levels			Blood Pressure Levels		Insulin/Medications		
Before:		Time:	(systolic):	Heart Rate (per min)	Type/Units	Pre	Post
After:		Time:	(diastolic):				

Snack #1

Totals:								

Blood Glucose Levels			Blood Pressure Levels		Insulin/Medications		
Before:		Time:	(systolic):	Heart Rate (per min)	Type/Units	Pre	Post
After:		Time:	(diastolic):				

Lunch

Totals:								

Blood Glucose Levels			Blood Pressure Levels		Insulin/Medications		
Before:		Time:	(systolic):	Heart Rate (per min)	Type/Units	Pre	Post
After:		Time:	(diastolic):				

Snack #2

Totals:								

Blood Glucose Levels			Blood Pressure Levels		Insulin/Medications		
Before:		Time:	(systolic):	Heart Rate (per min)	Type/Units	Pre	Post
After:		Time:	(diastolic):				

Dinner

Totals:								

Blood Glucose Levels			Blood Pressure Levels		Insulin/Medications		
Before:		Time:	(systolic):	Heart Rate (per min)	Type/Units	Pre	Post
After:		Time:	(diastolic):				

Fasting Blood Sugar:

_____

Water Intake:

total ounces _____

Fitness Log:

Activity	Min

Sleep Log:

Total Hours _____

Notes:

_____
_____
_____
_____
_____
_____
_____
_____
_____
_____

DAILY LOG

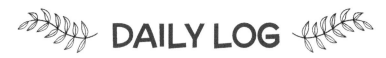

Date: ___/___/_____   **M T W Th F Sa Su**

Breakfast

	Meal	Calories	Fat (g)	Carbs (g)	Sugar (g)	Fiber (g)	Net Carb (carbs-fiber)	Protein (g)	Sodium (mg)
	Totals:								

Blood Glucose Levels			Blood Pressure Levels		Insulin/Medications		
Before:		Time:	(systolic):	Heart Rate (per min)	Type/Units	Pre	Post
After:		Time:	(diastolic):				

Snack #1

	Totals:								

Blood Glucose Levels			Blood Pressure Levels		Insulin/Medications		
Before:		Time:	(systolic):	Heart Rate (per min)	Type/Units	Pre	Post
After:		Time:	(diastolic):				

Lunch

	Totals:								

Blood Glucose Levels			Blood Pressure Levels		Insulin/Medications		
Before:		Time:	(systolic):	Heart Rate (per min)	Type/Units	Pre	Post
After:		Time:	(diastolic):				

Snack #2

	Totals:								

Blood Glucose Levels			Blood Pressure Levels		Insulin/Medications		
Before:		Time:	(systolic):	Heart Rate (per min)	Type/Units	Pre	Post
After:		Time:	(diastolic):				

Dinner

	Totals:								

Blood Glucose Levels			Blood Pressure Levels		Insulin/Medications		
Before:		Time:	(systolic):	Heart Rate (per min)	Type/Units	Pre	Post
After:		Time:	(diastolic):				

Fasting Blood Sugar:

_____

Water Intake:

total ounces _____

Fitness Log:

Activity	Min

Sleep Log:

Total Hours _____

Notes:

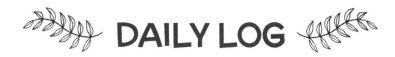

DAILY LOG

Date: ___/___/_____   **M T W Th F Sa Su**

Breakfast

Meal	Calories	Fat (g)	Carbs (g)	Sugar (g)	Fiber (g)	Net Carb (carbs-fiber)	Protein (g)	Sodium (mg)
Totals:								

Blood Glucose Levels			Blood Pressure Levels		Insulin/Medications		
Before:		Time:	(systolic):	Heart Rate (per min)	Type/Units	Pre	Post
After:		Time:	(diastolic):				

Snack #1

Totals:								

Blood Glucose Levels			Blood Pressure Levels		Insulin/Medications		
Before:		Time:	(systolic):	Heart Rate (per min)	Type/Units	Pre	Post
After:		Time:	(diastolic):				

Lunch

Totals:								

Blood Glucose Levels			Blood Pressure Levels		Insulin/Medications		
Before:		Time:	(systolic):	Heart Rate (per min)	Type/Units	Pre	Post
After:		Time:	(diastolic):				

Snack #2

Totals:								

Blood Glucose Levels			Blood Pressure Levels		Insulin/Medications		
Before:		Time:	(systolic):	Heart Rate (per min)	Type/Units	Pre	Post
After:		Time:	(diastolic):				

Dinner

Totals:								

Blood Glucose Levels			Blood Pressure Levels		Insulin/Medications		
Before:		Time:	(systolic):	Heart Rate (per min)	Type/Units	Pre	Post
After:		Time:	(diastolic):				

Fasting Blood Sugar:

_____

Water Intake:

🍶 🍶 🍶 🍶 🍶 🍶 🍶 🍶

total ounces _____

Fitness Log:

Activity   Min

Sleep Log:

Total Hours _____

Notes:

_____
_____
_____
_____
_____
_____
_____
_____
_____

DAILY LOG

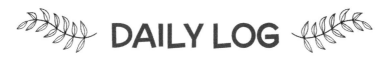

Date: ___/___/_____   **M T W Th F Sa Su**

Breakfast

Meal	Calories	Fat (g)	Carbs (g)	Sugar (g)	Fiber (g)	Net Carb (carbs-fiber)	Protein (g)	Sodium (mg)
Totals:								

Blood Glucose Levels			Blood Pressure Levels			Insulin/Medications		
Before:		Time:	(systolic):		Heart Rate (per min)	Type/Units	Pre	Post
After:		Time:	(diastolic):					

Fasting Blood Sugar:
_____

Water Intake:
total ounces _____

Snack #1

Totals:								

Blood Glucose Levels			Blood Pressure Levels			Insulin/Medications		
Before:		Time:	(systolic):		Heart Rate (per min)	Type/Units	Pre	Post
After:		Time:	(diastolic):					

Fitness Log:

Activity	Min

Lunch

Totals:								

Blood Glucose Levels			Blood Pressure Levels			Insulin/Medications		
Before:		Time:	(systolic):		Heart Rate (per min)	Type/Units	Pre	Post
After:		Time:	(diastolic):					

Sleep Log:
Total Hours _____

Snack #2

Totals:								

Blood Glucose Levels			Blood Pressure Levels			Insulin/Medications		
Before:		Time:	(systolic):		Heart Rate (per min)	Type/Units	Pre	Post
After:		Time:	(diastolic):					

Notes:
_____
_____
_____
_____
_____

Dinner

Totals:								

Blood Glucose Levels			Blood Pressure Levels			Insulin/Medications		
Before:		Time:	(systolic):		Heart Rate (per min)	Type/Units	Pre	Post
After:		Time:	(diastolic):					

DAILY LOG

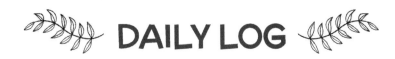

Date: ___/___/_____   **M T W Th F Sa Su**

Breakfast

	Meal	Calories	Fat (g)	Carbs (g)	Sugar (g)	Fiber (g)	Net Carb (carbs-fiber)	Protein (g)	Sodium (mg)
	Totals:								

Blood Glucose Levels				Blood Pressure Levels			Insulin/Medications		
Before:		Time:		(systolic):		Heart Rate (per min)	Type/Units	Pre	Post
After:		Time:		(diastolic):					

Snack #1

	Totals:								

Blood Glucose Levels				Blood Pressure Levels			Insulin/Medications		
Before:		Time:		(systolic):		Heart Rate (per min)	Type/Units	Pre	Post
After:		Time:		(diastolic):					

Lunch

	Totals:								

Blood Glucose Levels				Blood Pressure Levels			Insulin/Medications		
Before:		Time:		(systolic):		Heart Rate (per min)	Type/Units	Pre	Post
After:		Time:		(diastolic):					

Snack #2

	Totals:								

Blood Glucose Levels				Blood Pressure Levels			Insulin/Medications		
Before:		Time:		(systolic):		Heart Rate (per min)	Type/Units	Pre	Post
After:		Time:		(diastolic):					

Dinner

	Totals:								

Blood Glucose Levels				Blood Pressure Levels			Insulin/Medications		
Before:		Time:		(systolic):		Heart Rate (per min)	Type/Units	Pre	Post
After:		Time:		(diastolic):					

Fasting Blood Sugar:

_____

Water Intake:

total ounces _____

Fitness Log:

Activity	Min

Sleep Log:

Total Hours _____

Notes:

DAILY LOG

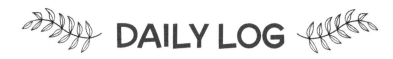

Date: ___/___/_____   **M T W Th F Sa Su**

Breakfast

Meal	Calories	Fat (g)	Carbs (g)	Sugar (g)	Fiber (g)	Net Carb (carbs-fiber)	Protein (g)	Sodium (mg)
Totals:								

Blood Glucose Levels				Blood Pressure Levels			Insulin/Medications		
Before:		Time:		(systolic):		Heart Rate (per min)	Type/Units	Pre	Post
After:		Time:		(diastolic):					

Snack #1

Totals:								

Blood Glucose Levels				Blood Pressure Levels			Insulin/Medications		
Before:		Time:		(systolic):		Heart Rate (per min)	Type/Units	Pre	Post
After:		Time:		(diastolic):					

Lunch

Totals:								

Blood Glucose Levels				Blood Pressure Levels			Insulin/Medications		
Before:		Time:		(systolic):		Heart Rate (per min)	Type/Units	Pre	Post
After:		Time:		(diastolic):					

Snack #2

Totals:								

Blood Glucose Levels				Blood Pressure Levels			Insulin/Medications		
Before:		Time:		(systolic):		Heart Rate (per min)	Type/Units	Pre	Post
After:		Time:		(diastolic):					

Dinner

Totals:								

Blood Glucose Levels				Blood Pressure Levels			Insulin/Medications		
Before:		Time:		(systolic):		Heart Rate (per min)	Type/Units	Pre	Post
After:		Time:		(diastolic):					

Fasting Blood Sugar:
_____

Water Intake:
🍼🍼🍼🍼🍼🍼🍼🍼
total ounces _____

Fitness Log:

Activity	Min

Sleep Log:
Total Hours _____

Notes:
_____
_____
_____
_____
_____
_____
_____
_____
_____
_____

DAILY LOG

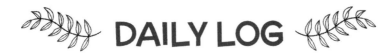

Date: ___/___/_____   **M T W Th F Sa Su**

Breakfast

Meal	Calories	Fat (g)	Carbs (g)	Sugar (g)	Fiber (g)	Net Carb (carbs-fiber)	Protein (g)	Sodium (mg)
Totals:								

Blood Glucose Levels		Blood Pressure Levels		Insulin/Medications		
Before:	Time:	(systolic):	Heart Rate (per min)	Type/Units	Pre	Post
After:	Time:	(diastolic):				

Snack #1

Totals:								

Blood Glucose Levels		Blood Pressure Levels		Insulin/Medications		
Before:	Time:	(systolic):	Heart Rate (per min)	Type/Units	Pre	Post
After:	Time:	(diastolic):				

Lunch

Totals:								

Blood Glucose Levels		Blood Pressure Levels		Insulin/Medications		
Before:	Time:	(systolic):	Heart Rate (per min)	Type/Units	Pre	Post
After:	Time:	(diastolic):				

Snack #2

Totals:								

Blood Glucose Levels		Blood Pressure Levels		Insulin/Medications		
Before:	Time:	(systolic):	Heart Rate (per min)	Type/Units	Pre	Post
After:	Time:	(diastolic):				

Dinner

Totals:								

Blood Glucose Levels		Blood Pressure Levels		Insulin/Medications		
Before:	Time:	(systolic):	Heart Rate (per min)	Type/Units	Pre	Post
After:	Time:	(diastolic):				

Fasting Blood Sugar:

_____

Water Intake:

total ounces _____

Fitness Log:

Activity	Min

Sleep Log:

Total Hours _____

Notes:

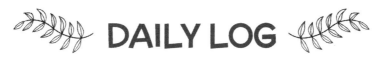

DAILY LOG

Date: ___/___/_____   **M T W Th F Sa Su**

Breakfast

	Meal	Calories	Fat (g)	Carbs (g)	Sugar (g)	Fiber (g)	Net Carb (carbs-fiber)	Protein (g)	Sodium (mg)
Totals:									

Blood Glucose Levels			Blood Pressure Levels		Heart Rate (per min)	Insulin/Medications		
Before:		Time:	(systolic):			Type/Units	Pre	Post
After:		Time:	(diastolic):					

Snack #1

Totals:									

Blood Glucose Levels			Blood Pressure Levels		Heart Rate (per min)	Insulin/Medications		
Before:		Time:	(systolic):			Type/Units	Pre	Post
After:		Time:	(diastolic):					

Lunch

Totals:									

Blood Glucose Levels			Blood Pressure Levels		Heart Rate (per min)	Insulin/Medications		
Before:		Time:	(systolic):			Type/Units	Pre	Post
After:		Time:	(diastolic):					

Snack #2

Totals:									

Blood Glucose Levels			Blood Pressure Levels		Heart Rate (per min)	Insulin/Medications		
Before:		Time:	(systolic):			Type/Units	Pre	Post
After:		Time:	(diastolic):					

Dinner

Totals:									

Blood Glucose Levels			Blood Pressure Levels		Heart Rate (per min)	Insulin/Medications		
Before:		Time:	(systolic):			Type/Units	Pre	Post
After:		Time:	(diastolic):					

Fasting Blood Sugar:

_____

Water Intake:

total ounces _____

Fitness Log:

Activity	Min

Sleep Log:

Total Hours _____

Notes:

_____
_____
_____
_____
_____
_____
_____
_____
_____

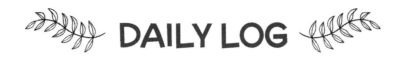

DAILY LOG

Date: ___/___/_____   **M T W Th F Sa Su**

Breakfast

Meal	Calories	Fat (g)	Carbs (g)	Sugar (g)	Fiber (g)	Net Carb (carbs-fiber)	Protein (g)	Sodium (mg)
Totals:								

Blood Glucose Levels			Blood Pressure Levels		Insulin/Medications		
Before:		Time:	(systolic):	Heart Rate (per min)	Type/Units	Pre	Post
After:		Time:	(diastolic):				

Fasting Blood Sugar:

_____

Snack #1

Meal	Calories	Fat (g)	Carbs (g)	Sugar (g)	Fiber (g)	Net Carb (carbs-fiber)	Protein (g)	Sodium (mg)
Totals:								

Blood Glucose Levels			Blood Pressure Levels		Insulin/Medications		
Before:		Time:	(systolic):	Heart Rate (per min)	Type/Units	Pre	Post
After:		Time:	(diastolic):				

Water Intake:

total ounces _____

Lunch

Meal	Calories	Fat (g)	Carbs (g)	Sugar (g)	Fiber (g)	Net Carb (carbs-fiber)	Protein (g)	Sodium (mg)
Totals:								

Blood Glucose Levels			Blood Pressure Levels		Insulin/Medications		
Before:		Time:	(systolic):	Heart Rate (per min)	Type/Units	Pre	Post
After:		Time:	(diastolic):				

Fitness Log:

Activity	Min

Sleep Log:

Total Hours _____

Snack #2

Meal	Calories	Fat (g)	Carbs (g)	Sugar (g)	Fiber (g)	Net Carb (carbs-fiber)	Protein (g)	Sodium (mg)
Totals:								

Blood Glucose Levels			Blood Pressure Levels		Insulin/Medications		
Before:		Time:	(systolic):	Heart Rate (per min)	Type/Units	Pre	Post
After:		Time:	(diastolic):				

Notes:

_____
_____
_____

Dinner

Meal	Calories	Fat (g)	Carbs (g)	Sugar (g)	Fiber (g)	Net Carb (carbs-fiber)	Protein (g)	Sodium (mg)
Totals:								

Blood Glucose Levels			Blood Pressure Levels		Insulin/Medications		
Before:		Time:	(systolic):	Heart Rate (per min)	Type/Units	Pre	Post
After:		Time:	(diastolic):				

DAILY LOG

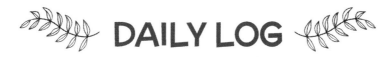

Date: ___/___/_____   **M T W Th F Sa Su**

Breakfast

	Meal	Calories	Fat (g)	Carbs (g)	Sugar (g)	Fiber (g)	Net Carb (carbs-fiber)	Protein (g)	Sodium (mg)
	Totals:								

Blood Glucose Levels			Blood Pressure Levels			Insulin/Medications		
Before:		Time:	(systolic):		Heart Rate (per min)	Type/Units	Pre	Post
After:		Time:	(diastolic):					

Snack #1

	Totals:								

Blood Glucose Levels			Blood Pressure Levels			Insulin/Medications		
Before:		Time:	(systolic):		Heart Rate (per min)	Type/Units	Pre	Post
After:		Time:	(diastolic):					

Lunch

	Totals:								

Blood Glucose Levels			Blood Pressure Levels			Insulin/Medications		
Before:		Time:	(systolic):		Heart Rate (per min)	Type/Units	Pre	Post
After:		Time:	(diastolic):					

Snack #2

	Totals:								

Blood Glucose Levels			Blood Pressure Levels			Insulin/Medications		
Before:		Time:	(systolic):		Heart Rate (per min)	Type/Units	Pre	Post
After:		Time:	(diastolic):					

Dinner

	Totals:								

Blood Glucose Levels			Blood Pressure Levels			Insulin/Medications		
Before:		Time:	(systolic):		Heart Rate (per min)	Type/Units	Pre	Post
After:		Time:	(diastolic):					

Fasting Blood Sugar:

_____

Water Intake:

🍼🍼🍼🍼🍼🍼🍼🍼

total ounces _____

Fitness Log:

Activity   Min

Sleep Log:

Total Hours _____

Notes:

_____
_____
_____
_____
_____
_____
_____
_____

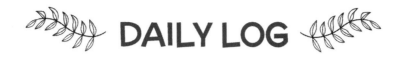

DAILY LOG

Date: ___/___/_____   **M T W Th F Sa Su**

Breakfast

Meal	Calories	Fat (g)	Carbs (g)	Sugar (g)	Fiber (g)	Net Carb (carbs-fiber)	Protein (g)	Sodium (mg)
Totals:								

Blood Glucose Levels			Blood Pressure Levels		Insulin/Medications		
Before:		Time:	(systolic):	Heart Rate (per min)	Type/Units	Pre	Post
After:		Time:	(diastolic):				

Snack #1

Totals:								

Blood Glucose Levels			Blood Pressure Levels		Insulin/Medications		
Before:		Time:	(systolic):	Heart Rate (per min)	Type/Units	Pre	Post
After:		Time:	(diastolic):				

Lunch

Totals:								

Blood Glucose Levels			Blood Pressure Levels		Insulin/Medications		
Before:		Time:	(systolic):	Heart Rate (per min)	Type/Units	Pre	Post
After:		Time:	(diastolic):				

Snack #2

Totals:								

Blood Glucose Levels			Blood Pressure Levels		Insulin/Medications		
Before:		Time:	(systolic):	Heart Rate (per min)	Type/Units	Pre	Post
After:		Time:	(diastolic):				

Dinner

Totals:								

Blood Glucose Levels			Blood Pressure Levels		Insulin/Medications		
Before:		Time:	(systolic):	Heart Rate (per min)	Type/Units	Pre	Post
After:		Time:	(diastolic):				

Fasting Blood Sugar:

_____

Water Intake:

total ounces _____

Fitness Log:

Activity	Min

Sleep Log:

Total Hours _____

Notes:

_____
_____
_____
_____
_____
_____
_____
_____
_____

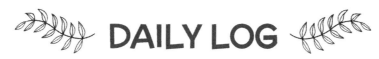

DAILY LOG

Date: ____/____/_____   **M T W Th F Sa Su**

Breakfast

Meal	Calories	Fat (g)	Carbs (g)	Sugar (g)	Fiber (g)	Net Carb (carbs-fiber)	Protein (g)	Sodium (mg)
Totals:								

Blood Glucose Levels			Blood Pressure Levels		Heart Rate (per min)	Insulin/Medications		
Before:		Time:	(systolic):			Type/Units	Pre	Post
After:		Time:	(diastolic):					

Fasting Blood Sugar:

_____

Snack #1

Totals:								

Blood Glucose Levels			Blood Pressure Levels		Heart Rate (per min)	Insulin/Medications		
Before:		Time:	(systolic):			Type/Units	Pre	Post
After:		Time:	(diastolic):					

Water Intake:

ὁὁὁὁὁὁὁὁ

total ounces _____

Lunch

Totals:								

Blood Glucose Levels			Blood Pressure Levels		Heart Rate (per min)	Insulin/Medications		
Before:		Time:	(systolic):			Type/Units	Pre	Post
After:		Time:	(diastolic):					

Fitness Log:

Activity	Min

Sleep Log:

Total Hours _____

Snack #2

Totals:								

Blood Glucose Levels			Blood Pressure Levels		Heart Rate (per min)	Insulin/Medications		
Before:		Time:	(systolic):			Type/Units	Pre	Post
After:		Time:	(diastolic):					

Notes:

Dinner

Totals:								

Blood Glucose Levels			Blood Pressure Levels		Heart Rate (per min)	Insulin/Medications		
Before:		Time:	(systolic):			Type/Units	Pre	Post
After:		Time:	(diastolic):					

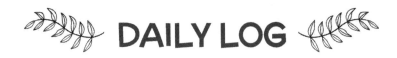

DAILY LOG

Date: ___/___/_____   **M T W Th F Sa Su**

Breakfast

Meal	Calories	Fat (g)	Carbs (g)	Sugar (g)	Fiber (g)	Net Carb (carbs-fiber)	Protein (g)	Sodium (mg)
Totals:								

Blood Glucose Levels				Blood Pressure Levels			Insulin/Medications		
Before:		Time:		(systolic):		Heart Rate (per min)	Type/Units	Pre	Post
After:		Time:		(diastolic):					

Snack #1

Meal	Calories	Fat (g)	Carbs (g)	Sugar (g)	Fiber (g)	Net Carb (carbs-fiber)	Protein (g)	Sodium (mg)
Totals:								

Blood Glucose Levels				Blood Pressure Levels			Insulin/Medications		
Before:		Time:		(systolic):		Heart Rate (per min)	Type/Units	Pre	Post
After:		Time:		(diastolic):					

Lunch

Meal	Calories	Fat (g)	Carbs (g)	Sugar (g)	Fiber (g)	Net Carb (carbs-fiber)	Protein (g)	Sodium (mg)
Totals:								

Blood Glucose Levels				Blood Pressure Levels			Insulin/Medications		
Before:		Time:		(systolic):		Heart Rate (per min)	Type/Units	Pre	Post
After:		Time:		(diastolic):					

Snack #2

Meal	Calories	Fat (g)	Carbs (g)	Sugar (g)	Fiber (g)	Net Carb (carbs-fiber)	Protein (g)	Sodium (mg)
Totals:								

Blood Glucose Levels				Blood Pressure Levels			Insulin/Medications		
Before:		Time:		(systolic):		Heart Rate (per min)	Type/Units	Pre	Post
After:		Time:		(diastolic):					

Dinner

Meal	Calories	Fat (g)	Carbs (g)	Sugar (g)	Fiber (g)	Net Carb (carbs-fiber)	Protein (g)	Sodium (mg)
Totals:								

Blood Glucose Levels				Blood Pressure Levels			Insulin/Medications		
Before:		Time:		(systolic):		Heart Rate (per min)	Type/Units	Pre	Post
After:		Time:		(diastolic):					

Fasting Blood Sugar:

_____

Water Intake:

total ounces _____

Fitness Log:

Activity	Min

Sleep Log:

Total Hours _____

Notes:

DAILY LOG

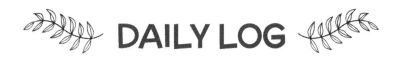

Date: ___/___/_____   **M T W Th F Sa Su**

Breakfast

	Meal	Calories	Fat (g)	Carbs (g)	Sugar (g)	Fiber (g)	Net Carb (carbs-fiber)	Protein (g)	Sodium (mg)
	Totals:								

Blood Glucose Levels			Blood Pressure Levels			Insulin/Medications		
Before:		Time:	(systolic):		Heart Rate (per min)	Type/Units	Pre	Post
After:		Time:	(diastolic):					

Snack #1

	Totals:								

Blood Glucose Levels			Blood Pressure Levels			Insulin/Medications		
Before:		Time:	(systolic):		Heart Rate (per min)	Type/Units	Pre	Post
After:		Time:	(diastolic):					

Lunch

	Totals:								

Blood Glucose Levels			Blood Pressure Levels			Insulin/Medications		
Before:		Time:	(systolic):		Heart Rate (per min)	Type/Units	Pre	Post
After:		Time:	(diastolic):					

Snack #2

	Totals:								

Blood Glucose Levels			Blood Pressure Levels			Insulin/Medications		
Before:		Time:	(systolic):		Heart Rate (per min)	Type/Units	Pre	Post
After:		Time:	(diastolic):					

Dinner

	Totals:								

Blood Glucose Levels			Blood Pressure Levels			Insulin/Medications		
Before:		Time:	(systolic):		Heart Rate (per min)	Type/Units	Pre	Post
After:		Time:	(diastolic):					

Fasting Blood Sugar:

_____

Water Intake:

total ounces _____

Fitness Log:

Activity	Min

Sleep Log:

Total Hours _____

Notes:

_____
_____
_____
_____
_____
_____
_____
_____
_____

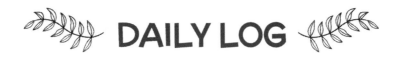

DAILY LOG

Date: ___/___/_____   M   T   W   Th   F   Sa   Su

Breakfast

Meal	Calories	Fat (g)	Carbs (g)	Sugar (g)	Fiber (g)	Net Carb (carbs-fiber)	Protein (g)	Sodium (mg)
Totals:								

Blood Glucose Levels			Blood Pressure Levels			Insulin/Medications		
Before:		Time:		(systolic):		Heart Rate (per min)	Type/Units	Pre	Post
After:		Time:		(diastolic):					

Snack #1

Totals:								

Blood Glucose Levels			Blood Pressure Levels			Insulin/Medications		
Before:		Time:		(systolic):		Heart Rate (per min)	Type/Units	Pre	Post
After:		Time:		(diastolic):					

Lunch

Totals:								

Blood Glucose Levels			Blood Pressure Levels			Insulin/Medications		
Before:		Time:		(systolic):		Heart Rate (per min)	Type/Units	Pre	Post
After:		Time:		(diastolic):					

Snack #2

Totals:								

Blood Glucose Levels			Blood Pressure Levels			Insulin/Medications		
Before:		Time:		(systolic):		Heart Rate (per min)	Type/Units	Pre	Post
After:		Time:		(diastolic):					

Dinner

Totals:								

Blood Glucose Levels			Blood Pressure Levels			Insulin/Medications		
Before:		Time:		(systolic):		Heart Rate (per min)	Type/Units	Pre	Post
After:		Time:		(diastolic):					

Fasting Blood Sugar:

_____

Water Intake:

total ounces _____

Fitness Log:

Activity	Min

Sleep Log:

Total Hours _____

Notes:

_____
_____
_____
_____
_____
_____

DAILY LOG

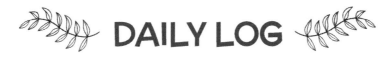

Date: ___/___/_____   **M   T   W   Th   F   Sa   Su**

Breakfast

Meal	Calories	Fat (g)	Carbs (g)	Sugar (g)	Fiber (g)	Net Carb (carbs-fiber)	Protein (g)	Sodium (mg)
Totals:								

Blood Glucose Levels			Blood Pressure Levels			Insulin/Medications		
Before:		Time:	(systolic):		Heart Rate (per min)	Type/Units	Pre	Post
After:		Time:	(diastolic):					

Snack #1

Totals:								

Blood Glucose Levels			Blood Pressure Levels			Insulin/Medications		
Before:		Time:	(systolic):		Heart Rate (per min)	Type/Units	Pre	Post
After:		Time:	(diastolic):					

Lunch

Totals:								

Blood Glucose Levels			Blood Pressure Levels			Insulin/Medications		
Before:		Time:	(systolic):		Heart Rate (per min)	Type/Units	Pre	Post
After:		Time:	(diastolic):					

Snack #2

Totals:								

Blood Glucose Levels			Blood Pressure Levels			Insulin/Medications		
Before:		Time:	(systolic):		Heart Rate (per min)	Type/Units	Pre	Post
After:		Time:	(diastolic):					

Dinner

Totals:								

Blood Glucose Levels			Blood Pressure Levels			Insulin/Medications		
Before:		Time:	(systolic):		Heart Rate (per min)	Type/Units	Pre	Post
After:		Time:	(diastolic):					

Fasting Blood Sugar:
_____

Water Intake:
total ounces _____

Fitness Log:
Activity	Min

Sleep Log:
Total Hours _____

Notes:
_____
_____
_____
_____
_____
_____
_____
_____
_____
_____
_____

DAILY LOG

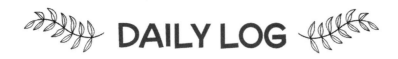

Date: ___/___/_____   **M T W Th F Sa Su**

Breakfast

Meal	Calories	Fat (g)	Carbs (g)	Sugar (g)	Fiber (g)	Net Carb (carbs-fiber)	Protein (g)	Sodium (mg)
Totals:								

Blood Glucose Levels				Blood Pressure Levels			Insulin/Medications		
Before:		Time:		(systolic):		Heart Rate (per min)	Type/Units	Pre	Post
After:		Time:		(diastolic):					

Snack #1

Totals:								

Blood Glucose Levels				Blood Pressure Levels			Insulin/Medications		
Before:		Time:		(systolic):		Heart Rate (per min)	Type/Units	Pre	Post
After:		Time:		(diastolic):					

Lunch

Totals:								

Blood Glucose Levels				Blood Pressure Levels			Insulin/Medications		
Before:		Time:		(systolic):		Heart Rate (per min)	Type/Units	Pre	Post
After:		Time:		(diastolic):					

Snack #2

Totals:								

Blood Glucose Levels				Blood Pressure Levels			Insulin/Medications		
Before:		Time:		(systolic):		Heart Rate (per min)	Type/Units	Pre	Post
After:		Time:		(diastolic):					

Dinner

Totals:								

Blood Glucose Levels				Blood Pressure Levels			Insulin/Medications		
Before:		Time:		(systolic):		Heart Rate (per min)	Type/Units	Pre	Post
After:		Time:		(diastolic):					

Fasting Blood Sugar:

_____

Water Intake:

total ounces _____

Fitness Log:

Activity	Min

Sleep Log:

Total Hours _____

Notes:

_____
_____
_____
_____
_____
_____
_____
_____

DAILY LOG

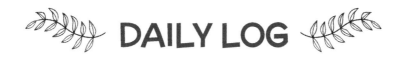

Date: ___/___/_____   **M T W Th F Sa Su**

Breakfast

Meal	Calories	Fat (g)	Carbs (g)	Sugar (g)	Fiber (g)	Net Carb (carbs-fiber)	Protein (g)	Sodium (mg)
Totals:								

Blood Glucose Levels			Blood Pressure Levels			Insulin/Medications		
Before:		Time:	(systolic):		Heart Rate (per min)	Type/Units	Pre	Post
After:		Time:	(diastolic):					

Snack #1

Totals:								

Blood Glucose Levels			Blood Pressure Levels			Insulin/Medications		
Before:		Time:	(systolic):		Heart Rate (per min)	Type/Units	Pre	Post
After:		Time:	(diastolic):					

Lunch

Totals:								

Blood Glucose Levels			Blood Pressure Levels			Insulin/Medications		
Before:		Time:	(systolic):		Heart Rate (per min)	Type/Units	Pre	Post
After:		Time:	(diastolic):					

Snack #2

Totals:								

Blood Glucose Levels			Blood Pressure Levels			Insulin/Medications		
Before:		Time:	(systolic):		Heart Rate (per min)	Type/Units	Pre	Post
After:		Time:	(diastolic):					

Dinner

Totals:								

Blood Glucose Levels			Blood Pressure Levels			Insulin/Medications		
Before:		Time:	(systolic):		Heart Rate (per min)	Type/Units	Pre	Post
After:		Time:	(diastolic):					

Fasting Blood Sugar:

_____

Water Intake:

total ounces _____

Fitness Log:

Activity	Min

Sleep Log:

Total Hours _____

Notes:

_____
_____
_____
_____
_____
_____
_____
_____
_____
_____
_____

DAILY LOG

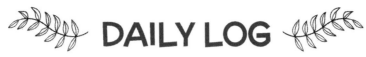

Date: ___/___/_____   **M   T   W   Th   F   Sa   Su**

Breakfast

Meal	Calories	Fat (g)	Carbs (g)	Sugar (g)	Fiber (g)	Net Carb (carbs-fiber)	Protein (g)	Sodium (mg)
Totals:								

Blood Glucose Levels			Blood Pressure Levels			Insulin/Medications		
			(systolic):		Heart Rate (per min)	Type/Units	Pre	Post
Before:		Time:						
After:		Time:	(diastolic):					

Snack #1

Meal	Calories	Fat (g)	Carbs (g)	Sugar (g)	Fiber (g)	Net Carb (carbs-fiber)	Protein (g)	Sodium (mg)
Totals:								

Blood Glucose Levels			Blood Pressure Levels			Insulin/Medications		
			(systolic):		Heart Rate (per min)	Type/Units	Pre	Post
Before:		Time:						
After:		Time:	(diastolic):					

Lunch

Meal	Calories	Fat (g)	Carbs (g)	Sugar (g)	Fiber (g)	Net Carb (carbs-fiber)	Protein (g)	Sodium (mg)
Totals:								

Blood Glucose Levels			Blood Pressure Levels			Insulin/Medications		
			(systolic):		Heart Rate (per min)	Type/Units	Pre	Post
Before:		Time:						
After:		Time:	(diastolic):					

Snack #2

Meal	Calories	Fat (g)	Carbs (g)	Sugar (g)	Fiber (g)	Net Carb (carbs-fiber)	Protein (g)	Sodium (mg)
Totals:								

Blood Glucose Levels			Blood Pressure Levels			Insulin/Medications		
			(systolic):		Heart Rate (per min)	Type/Units	Pre	Post
Before:		Time:						
After:		Time:	(diastolic):					

Dinner

Meal	Calories	Fat (g)	Carbs (g)	Sugar (g)	Fiber (g)	Net Carb (carbs-fiber)	Protein (g)	Sodium (mg)
Totals:								

Blood Glucose Levels			Blood Pressure Levels			Insulin/Medications		
			(systolic):		Heart Rate (per min)	Type/Units	Pre	Post
Before:		Time:						
After:		Time:	(diastolic):					

Fasting Blood Sugar:

_____

Water Intake:

🍶 🍶 🍶 🍶 🍶 🍶 🍶 🍶

total ounces _____

Fitness Log:

Activity	Min

Sleep Log:

Total Hours _____

Notes:

_____
_____
_____
_____
_____
_____
_____
_____
_____
_____

DAILY LOG

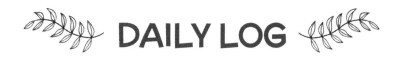

Date: ___/___/_____   **M T W Th F Sa Su**

Breakfast

Meal	Calories	Fat (g)	Carbs (g)	Sugar (g)	Fiber (g)	Net Carb (carbs-fiber)	Protein (g)	Sodium (mg)
Totals:								

Blood Glucose Levels			Blood Pressure Levels			Insulin/Medications		
Before:		Time:	(systolic):		Heart Rate (per min)	Type/Units	Pre	Post
After:		Time:	(diastolic):					

Snack #1

Totals:								

Blood Glucose Levels			Blood Pressure Levels			Insulin/Medications		
Before:		Time:	(systolic):		Heart Rate (per min)	Type/Units	Pre	Post
After:		Time:	(diastolic):					

Lunch

Totals:								

Blood Glucose Levels			Blood Pressure Levels			Insulin/Medications		
Before:		Time:	(systolic):		Heart Rate (per min)	Type/Units	Pre	Post
After:		Time:	(diastolic):					

Snack #2

Totals:								

Blood Glucose Levels			Blood Pressure Levels			Insulin/Medications		
Before:		Time:	(systolic):		Heart Rate (per min)	Type/Units	Pre	Post
After:		Time:	(diastolic):					

Dinner

Totals:								

Blood Glucose Levels			Blood Pressure Levels			Insulin/Medications		
Before:		Time:	(systolic):		Heart Rate (per min)	Type/Units	Pre	Post
After:		Time:	(diastolic):					

Fasting Blood Sugar:

_____

Water Intake:

total ounces _____

Fitness Log:

Activity	Min

Sleep Log:

Total Hours _____

Notes:

_____
_____
_____
_____
_____
_____
_____
_____
_____
_____
_____

DAILY LOG
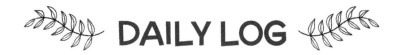

Date: ___/___/_____   M T W Th F Sa Su

Breakfast

Meal	Calories	Fat (g)	Carbs (g)	Sugar (g)	Fiber (g)	Net Carb (carbs-fiber)	Protein (g)	Sodium (mg)
Totals:								

Blood Glucose Levels			Blood Pressure Levels			Insulin/Medications		
Before:		Time:	(systolic):		Heart Rate (per min)	Type/Units	Pre	Post
After:		Time:	(diastolic):					

Snack #1

Totals:								

Blood Glucose Levels			Blood Pressure Levels			Insulin/Medications		
Before:		Time:	(systolic):		Heart Rate (per min)	Type/Units	Pre	Post
After:		Time:	(diastolic):					

Lunch

Totals:								

Blood Glucose Levels			Blood Pressure Levels			Insulin/Medications		
Before:		Time:	(systolic):		Heart Rate (per min)	Type/Units	Pre	Post
After:		Time:	(diastolic):					

Snack #2

Totals:								

Blood Glucose Levels			Blood Pressure Levels			Insulin/Medications		
Before:		Time:	(systolic):		Heart Rate (per min)	Type/Units	Pre	Post
After:		Time:	(diastolic):					

Dinner

Totals:								

Blood Glucose Levels			Blood Pressure Levels			Insulin/Medications		
Before:		Time:	(systolic):		Heart Rate (per min)	Type/Units	Pre	Post
After:		Time:	(diastolic):					

Fasting Blood Sugar:

_____

Water Intake:

total ounces _____

Fitness Log:

Activity	Min

Sleep Log:

Total Hours _____

Notes:

_____
_____
_____
_____
_____
_____
_____
_____
_____

Made in United States
Troutdale, OR
09/17/2023

12990915R00108